Lipedema

Zaher Jandali • Lucian P. Jiga
Corrado Campisi
Editors

Lipedema

A Practical Guidebook

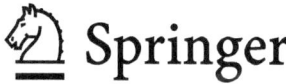 Springer

Editors
Zaher Jandali
Department of Plastic, Aesthetic
Reconstructive and Hand Surgery
Evangelical Hospital Oldenburg
26131 Oldenburg, Niedersachsen
Germany

Lucian P. Jiga
Department of Plastic, Aesthetic
Reconstructive and Hand Surgery
Evangelical Hospital Oldenburg
26131 Oldenburg, Niedersachsen
Germany

Corrado Campisi
ICLAS -Rapallo
GVM Care & Research
Genova
Italy

Translation from the German language edition: Lipödem und Lymphödem by Lucian P. Jiga, et al., © Springer-Verlag GmbH Deutschland, ein Teil von Springer Nature 2021. Published by Springer Berlin Heidelberg. All Rights Reserved.

ISBN 978-3-030-86716-4   ISBN 978-3-030-86717-1   (eBook)
https://doi.org/10.1007/978-3-030-86717-1

This Springer imprint is published by the registered company Springer Nature Switzerland AG
The registered company address is: Gewerbestrasse 11, 6330 Cham, Switzerland

Preface

Many women suffer from a painful disproportional tissue distribution in the extremities, especially the legs, and often know that something is wrong with them long before being diagnosed. It is the pain in the legs and arms that leads those affected to embark on a sometimes adventurous search for a diagnosis and possible ways for medical treatment. Lipedema is often misdiagnosed, so usually patients will have to change several doctors before finally confronted with the real diagnosis. As a rule, the first question most of the patients ask after being diagnosed is how the treatment looks like and how long will it take. Ignorance about the condition often fuels fears that the condition will progress rapidly without being able to do anything to stop it. These in turn will have an important negative effect on the patient's well-being but also generate a major psychological burden affecting the self-esteem and social relations. Aesthetics also play an important role that should not be underestimated.

Although knowledge about the disease "lipedema" has improved significantly in recent years, especially since entire health systems have considered giving it more attention, it is often based on incorrect information, assumptions, and facts. One thing is certain: there is a general lack of information on the subject of lipedema. This starts with the scientific side, continues with the specialized knowledge, and ends with the treatment, whether conservative or surgical. Therefore, it is important to us that we approach the topic of "lipedema" systematically and illuminate it from all aspects.

We hope, through this book, to offer at least a small contribution towards a much better understanding of this complex disease. Irrespective of this, professional societies, physicians, and centers must continue to work on transparency and knowledge transfer on all fronts in the future. Only in this way can we come closer to the goal of providing the best possible care for those affected.

With this book, we would like to provide those affected by lipedema with a practical guide.

We wish you an informative read.

Niedersachsen, Germany   Zaher Jandali
Niedersachsen, Germany   Lucian Jiga
Genova, Italy   Corrado Campisi

The Rationale for the Book

The idea for the book had been floating around in our minds for a long time, but as is often the case, there is simply not enough time to implement such projects.

The idea finally took form during one of the yearly meetings we organized for our colleagues for education and training in the field of lymphatic and lipedema surgery. I remember well when we talked about the poor transfer of knowledge to those affected. It doesn't even start with the patients; it starts with us, the physicians! There are many colleagues who have never heard of lipedema or lymphedema and are not familiar with the differentiation between these two conditions. What level of knowledge should the patients have about this disease?

At the same time, talking about our scientific projects we found out that we do a lot in the field of lymphatic surgery, but quite little to nothing in the field of lipedema, although this issue accounts for a much larger share in our clinical routine. Furthermore, contemplating the actual evidence on lipedema we identified a major gap in both medical and patient-oriented literature.

Our motivation for this book was to convey the current state of scientific knowledge in terms understandable for our patients and everyone interested to learn more about this condition.

Acknowledgements

Most readers see the editors and authors as the creators of a book. As this might be true for the idea and content, completing such a task takes much more than these to achieve. As such, we would like to thank all who helped and supported us from the bottom of our hearts starting with our patients who offered us their unbounded trust, motivating us to write this book. For us, it is a matter of the heart to help patients affected with lipedema.

We would like to thank Mrs. Jandali and Mr. Stober (www.svenstober.com) for the great pictures, with the help of which readers will definitely get a much better view of the individual explanations throughout the book.

We owe a big thank you to Springer, who believed in our idea and recognized the need for this book. Special mention should be made of the project planner Ms. Kraplow and project manager Ms. Beisel. We have rarely experienced such dedicated cooperation.

Very special thanks go to our proofreader Mrs. Thürk. From the first moment of cooperation, we felt very well taken care of. The proofreading made the book an easy lecture, giving it a great boost. Thank you for your patience with us. It was certainly a difficult task, which you mastered brilliantly.

About this Book

The idea to write this book was fueled from many years of experience in dealing with affected patients and their families. With this book, we have set ourselves the goal of giving the reader an in-depth overview on all aspects related to "lipedema" helping you to make your own treatment decisions.

At the beginning of the book, the current scientific knowledge is summarized. In doing so, we dispel many half-truths and myths. In a structured way, the cause of lipedema, its clinical picture, and how this disease manifests itself are explained. Finally, its consequences as well as supposedly similar diseases such as pure lymph-edema and obesity are discussed. Furthermore, we discuss the current classification we use of lipedema as we would like it to be.

We then enter into our actual core topic, the treatment of lipedema. In addition to the aspects of the timing of a treatment, we deal with the different conservative and surgical options. At the end, we provide the reader with our recommendations for treatment.

All the above are of course only rough headings of the topics that await you in this book. Look forward to exciting details and in-depth expertise to help you sharpen your view on the topic of "lipedema."

After reading this book you will be familiar with all actual treatment options for lipedema. In particular, through the information you will discover in this book, you will be given the chance to weigh up the advantages and disadvantages of each individual procedure according to your own symptoms. We are confident that by reading this guide, your level of knowledge and your self-confidence will increase, making the next visit to your doctor a "walk in the park" instead of a chaotic uncontrolled input of unknown information.

However, this book is neither thought as a substitute for a doctor appointment and since medicine is in a constant state of development nor as a complete or up to date reference for lipedema. Likewise, each chapter reflects the opinion of its respective authors.

This book is NOT a scientific publication. It targets mainly the "non-medical readership," who by reading it should gain a thorough understanding of this painful fat tissue disease.

No before-and-after pictures of operations are shown in this book, so as not to give the impression that advertising for surgical measures is being carried out. If before-and-after images are shown, they are 3D illustrations and not actual images.

Enjoy reading.

Contents

1 The Lipedema 1

Zaher Jandali, Benedikt Merwart, and Lucian Jiga

1.1 Introduction 1

1.2 Causes and Emergence. 4

    1.2.1 Adipose Tissue. 5

    1.2.2 Science in Detail 9

    1.2.3 Hormone Activity of the Adipose Tissue 12

    1.2.4 Lipohypertrophy 17

    1.2.5 Theory of Microvascular Disruption and Lymphatic Interaction 21

    1.2.6 Uncontrolled Fat Tissue Proliferation 21

1.3 The Edema. 23

1.4 Pain 30

1.5 A Chronic-Progressive Course?. 31

1.6 Obesity and Lipedema. 32

1.7 Complaints and Effects of Lipedema. 44

1.8 Appearance, Stages, Classifications, and Course. 48

1.9 Diagnosis 56

2 The Lymphedema 69

Corrado Campisi, Lucian Jiga, and Zaher Jandali

2.1 Anatomy and Functioning of the Lymphatic System 69

2.2 Causes 73

2.3 Clinical Appearance. 75

2.4 Diagnosis 76

2.5 Conservative Therapy 78

2.6 Surgical Therapy 81

    2.6.1 Restorative/Reconstructive Surgery. 82

    2.6.2 Tissue Removal Measures 85

2.7 Similarities and Differences of Lipedema and Lymphedema 88

3   Treatment of Lipedema 95
      Zaher Jandali, Benedikt Merwart, Ralf Weise, Angel Pecorelli
      Capozzi, and Lucian Jiga
      3.1   Introduction 95
      3.2   Measures for Weight Stabilization.......................... 98
             3.2.1   Conservative Measures 98
             3.2.2   Surgical Measures for Weight Stabilization............. 101
      3.3   Complex Physical Therapy 107
      3.4   Complex Surgical Treatment 111
      3.5   The Individual Therapy Plan 114
      3.6   The Liposuction 115
             3.6.1   General Information.............................. 115
             3.6.2   Techniques and Shapes 117
             3.6.3   Liposuction Volume 123
      3.7   Conclusion 130
             3.7.1   Requirements and Preparations 130
             3.7.2   Liposuction Procedure............................ 136
             3.7.3   Aftercare 140
             3.7.4   Success and Long-Term Prospects.................... 146
             3.7.5   Consequences and Risks 150
             3.7.6   Course of the Complex-Operative Therapy Plan.......... 160
      3.8   Treatment Example 166
      3.9   Cost Absorption 167
      3.10   Autologous Fat Grafting 171

**4   Body Contouring Surgery After Extensive Liposuction
      and Weight Loss** 177
      Zaher Jandali, Benedikt Merwart, and Lucian Jiga
      4.1   Medical Indication for Tightening of Excess Skin
             and Soft Tissues....................................... 177
      4.2   Noninvasive and Minimally Invasive Tightening Methods 178
      4.3   Conclusion 180
      4.4   Thigh Lift.. 181
      4.5   Upper Arm Lift 186
      4.6   Buttock Lift 190
      4.7   Tightening of the Lower Torso Wall 191

5   Additional Information about Treatment...................... 199
      Zaher Jandali, Benedikt Merwart, and Lucian Jiga
      5.1   Possibilities and Limits of Plastic Surgery 199
      5.2   How to Find the Right Doctor? 200
      5.3   Presentation to the Plastic Surgeon 201

Index.. 205

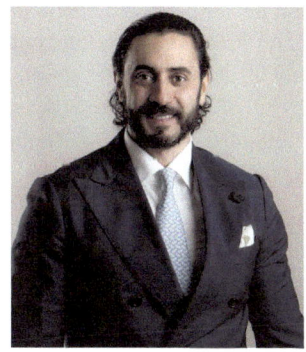

Corrado Campisi, MD, Ph.D., MRM is a plastic, reconstructive, and aesthetic surgeon based in Genoa, Italy (GVM Care & Research: ICLAS—Rapallo, Genoa; Salus Hospital—Reggio Emilia; Maria Pia Hospital—Turin), and an Adjunct Professor of Plastic Surgery at the University of Catania, Italy. He completed his Ph.D. in Experimental Surgery and Microsurgery at the University of Pavia, Italy, and his Master's Degree in Reconstructive Microsurgery at the UAB in Barcelona, Spain (Reconstructive Microsurgery European School—RMES). He is an Executive Committee Member of the International Society of Lymphology (ISL) and will host the 23rd ISL World Congress in Turin in 2023. He has published numerous scientific papers and contributed to several books on the surgical treatment of lymphedema. The Genoa Lymphedema Clinic is internationally known and receives patients from all over the world.

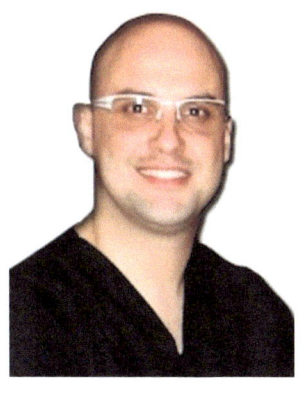

Angel Pecorelli Capozzi, M.D. is a specialist in plastic and reconstructive surgery. Dr. Pecorelli completed his undergraduate and six-year residency in Venezuela. Three years of his six-year residency were in the Department of Oral and Maxillofacial Surgery at the Dr. Miguel Perez Carreño Clinic, Caracas-Venezuela. Dr. Pecorelli completed his postgraduate studies with a focus on aesthetic and noninvasive treatments and physiological aging medicine. Dr. Pecorelli is the owner of Platinum Medical Center in Barcelona, Spain. Plastic & Reconstructive Surgery Specialist Specialization Postgraduate in Cosmetic & Aesthetic Medicine Specialization

Postgraduate in Physiological Aging Medicine Member of the Ibero-Latin American Federation of Plastic Surgery (FILACP) Member of the Venezuelan Society of Plastic Reconstructive Aesthetic and Maxillo-Facial Surgery (SVCPREM) CEO at Platinum Medical Center (Barcelona, Spain) Board of Director of Spanish Society of Facial Plastic Surgery (SECPF) Vice-President of the Latin-American Society of Facial Aesthetic Surgery (SOLAFACE) International Educator in the Spanish Society of Facial Plastic Surgery (SECPF) Member of the Spanish Society of Cosmetic Surgery and Medicine (SEMCC) E-Mail: pecorellicapozziad@icloud.com Web: www.platinumbarcelona.com

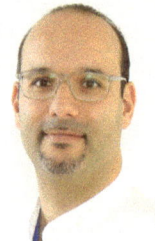

Zaher Jandali, M.D. graduated in 2006 at the University Medical Center Hamburg-Eppendorf (UKE) in Hamburg as medical doctor. In 2012 he completed his training as consultant in plastic and aesthetic surgery in the Department of Plastic, Aesthetic, Reconstructive and Hand Surgery at the Asklepios Clinic in Hamburg-Wandsbek. Since day one, Dr. Jandali has been intensively involved with the topic of "lipedema." Early on, he began giving lectures to those affected and interested, as well as to patient support groups. This was followed by lectures on this topic at national and international congresses. Since 2016, Dr. Jandali occupies the chair position of the Clinic for Plastic, Reconstructive, Aesthetic and Hand Surgery at the Evangelical Hospital in Oldenburg (Lower Saxony). Dr. Jandali further developed several surgical techniques for lipedema, combining different approaches to achieve better and safer results. Since 2007, his main focus has been on the treatment of lipedema and lymphedema. He performs liposuction using a unique technique optimized for lipedema. Dr. Jandali also focuses on reconstructive surgery after weight loss, as well as aesthetic and reconstructive microsurgery. Dr. Jandali is a member of the following professional societies: DGPRÄC, German Society of Plastic, Reconstructive and Aesthetic Surgeons DGH, German Society for Hand Surgery WSRM, World Society of Reconstructive Microsurgery www.jandali.de www.lipold.de

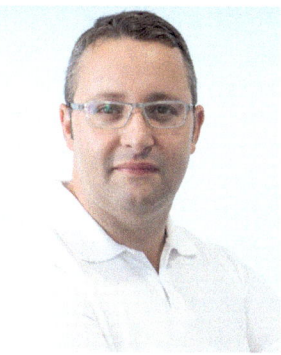

Lucian Jiga, M.D. completed his medical studies at the Victor Babes University of Medicine and Pharmacy Timisoara in Romania. In 2002, he moved to the Ruprecht-Karls-University of Heidelberg for pursuing a research fellowship that led him to successfully defend his doctoral thesis three years later. After his stay in Heidelberg, in 2005 Dr. Jiga moved back to Timisoara to the University Clinic for Vascular Surgery and Reconstructive Microsurgery. Starting in 2009, he occupied the section chair position as Associate Professor in the Department of Reconstructive Microsurgery. In 2013, Dr. Jiga returned to Germany as a senior consultant of the Clinic for Plastic, Aesthetic, Reconstructive and Hand Surgery at the Evangelisches Krankenhaus in Oldenburg. Since 2016 he shares here the chair of department position with Dr. Jandali. Dr. Jiga looks back on a large number of international lectures and scientific publications. In addition to the treatment of lipedema, his clinical work focuses on reconstructive surgery after breast cancer and after weight loss, the treatment of lymphedema, microsurgical reconstructive surgery, especially to preserve extremities, and complex hand surgery. Dr. Jiga is a member of the following professional societies: DGPRÄC, German Society of Plastic, Reconstructive and Aesthetic Surgeons DGH, German Society for Hand Surgery WSRM, World Society of Reconstructive Microsurgery TTS, The Transplantation Society.

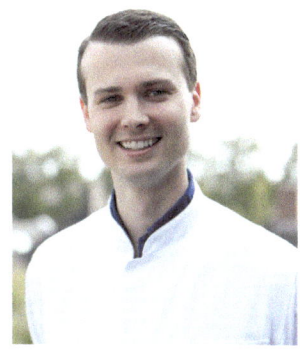

Benedikt Merwart completed his medical studies at Heinrich Heine University in Düsseldorf, Germany, graduating in 2015. He discovered his interest in the treatment and therapy of lipedema and lymphedema early on in his training, which he began in 2015 at the Clinic for Plastic, Aesthetic, Reconstructive and Hand Surgery at the Evangelisches Krankenhaus under the direction of Dr. med. Z. Jandali and Dr. med. L.P. Jiga. Mr. Merwart regularly lectures on this topic for affected individuals and self-help groups as well as at national and international professional congresses. His other areas of interest include breast reconstruction after breast cancer treatment and restoration of body shape after massive weight loss. Mr. Merwart is the author of several scientific publications and books.

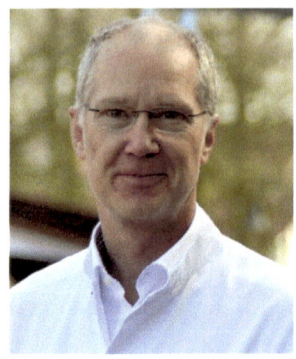

Ralf Weise, M.D. is a specialist in general, visceral and special visceral surgery, a specialist in surgical proctology, certified in minimally invasive surgery (CAMIC), and a specialist in nutritional medicine. Since 2006, he has been the head physician of the Clinic for General and Visceral Surgery at St.-Marien-Hospital in Friesoythe. In 2007, he founded the North-West Obesity Center, which was certified as a Center of Excellence in 2011 and as a Reference Center in 2015. In 2017, the Obesity Center celebrated its 10th anniversary. To date, more than 3,500 obese patients have been treated in Friesoythe and more than 1,700 metabolic interventions have been performed. Dr. Weise has served as medical director at St.-Marien-Hospital in Friesoythe since 2013. He has given numerous lectures and presentations at international congresses and has published articles on obesity in four books. www.weiseoperiert.de www.adipositas-zentrum-nord-west.de

The Lipedema

Zaher Jandali, Benedikt Merwart, and Lucian Jiga

1.1 Introduction

Lipedema is recognized as a disease, yet it is trivialized by many colleagues, frequently being used as a "way out diagnosis," according to the motto: "If we don't find anything and you have thick legs, then you have lipedema." Patients with lipedema suffer from a serious illness that is responsible for significant suffering. The complex clinical picture of lipedema cannot simply be reduced to painful legs and arms. It cannot be equated with "thick legs" or "thick arms," nor can all thick legs and arms be attributed to lipedema. It is therefore important to make an accurate diagnosis clearly distinguishing lipedema from other diseases (Fig. 1.1).

Perhaps you are a patient yourself, with high hopes of being cured, reading this book to learn more about your disease. If so, you match the profile of the majority of patients addressing us for possible treatment. Unfortunately, after their first appointment, most of these patients are faced with the fact that such expectations are sometimes far from what is actually possible. Either social media or physicians often fuel such discrepancies. Particularly inexperienced colleagues allow themselves, as a display of unsustainable knowledge "in front of the camera," to bring the topic "lipedema" into the public eye with questionable advances just for the sake of media attention. Despite several existing claims on lipedema being a curable disease, there is, unfortunately, no cure for it to date. However, with the right measures, the suffering can be sustainably alleviated and quality of life restored.

We have deliberately chosen these provocative introductory words to draw attention to the lack of acceptance of "lipedema" as a disease. If you really want to understand lipedema, you first have to find out the state of knowledge about this disease. Thus, we would first briefly discuss the history and origin of the term "lipedema."

Z. Jandali (✉) · B. Merwart · L. Jiga
Department of Plastic, Aesthetic, Reconstructive and Hand Surgery, Evangelical Hospital Oldenburg, Oldenburg, Niedersachsen, Germany
e-mail: dr@jandali.de

© Springer Nature Switzerland AG 2022
Z. Jandali et al. (eds.), *Lipedema*, https://doi.org/10.1007/978-3-030-86717-1_1

Fig. 1.1 Typical clinical
picture of moderately
pronounced lipedema

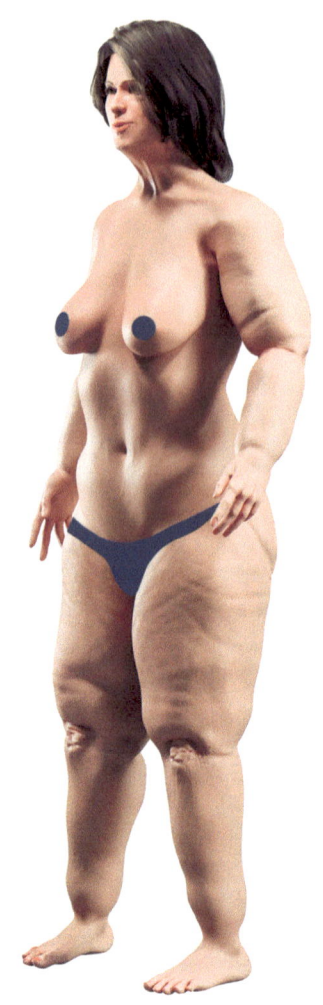

The Term "Lipedema"

The term "lipedema" comes from the ancient Greek term "fat swelling." It is composed of the two words λίπος, lípos, "fat" and the word οἴδημα, oídēma, "swelling." Synonyms for the term lipedema include pillar leg, lipalgia, adipoalgia, lipo-fat disease, lipohypertrophia dolorosa, and adiposity dolorosa of the arms and legs. In addition to these synonyms, there are many other terms of the same category that should NOT be used either because having a different meaning or no meaning at all. The examples are lipohypertrophy, breeches syndrome, lipidosis, fat-leg syndrome, lipdem, fatty leg, hyperplasia dolorosa, lipohyperplasia dolorosa, zonal obesity, and others (Table 1.1). Several of these terms will be explained in the book, as they are directly related to lipedema or should be distinguished from it.

Table 1.1 Actual and apparent synonyms of lipedema

Actual synonym	Apparent synonym
Painful column leg	Fat leg
Lipalgia	Lipdema, lipidosis
Adipoalgia, Adipoalgesia	Fat-leg syndrome
Lipohypertrophia dolorosa	Lipohypertrophy
Obesity dolorosa	Lipohyperplasia dolorosa
Painful lipedema syndrome	Hyperplasia dolorosa
Adiposis dolorosa	Zonal obesity

> ▶ We have long advocated abandoning the term lipedema and using the simple umbrella term "adipose tissue disease" with the sub-terms "lipalgia" or the term we introduced, "lipodolorosa (chronica)."

History of the Disease

Let us first look back at the history of the disease "lipedema" and what we have learned from the past. The first ones to describe lipedema were the physicians E.V. Allen and E.H. Hines in 1940 publishing the first scientific texts on the subject of "lipedema" in 1940, 1951, and 1952. Many scientific papers, websites and colleagues still refer to the rather old first descriptions. We roughly summarize the studies below to reflect their core statements.

The first of the three publications from 1940 is entitled "Lipedema of the legs: a syndrome characterized by fat legs and orthostatic edema" and describes a clinical syndrome that is often very distressing for those affected and could only be observed in women. Accordingly, the main complaints were swelling and an increase in adipose tissue volume and water retention in the area of the buttocks and legs. The swelling below the knee joint occurs predominantly when one is on one's feet a lot or during warm weather. Pain in the legs is also common. Furthermore, the syndrome is associated with a gradual increase in body weight. Unlike obesity, in which food intake exceeds the body's caloric needs, the increase in subcutaneous fat only on the buttocks and legs is not easily explained. The edema of the affected persons results from a passage of fluid from the blood into the tissue. If there was a fat distribution disorder in favor of the lower extremities without obesity, dietary measures would have no chance of success.

The second publication from 1951 with the very similar title "Lipedema of the legs; a syndrome characterized by fat legs and edema" describes lipedema as a progressive disease with orthostatic swelling of the legs. Compared to lymphedema, a decrease in leg swelling will not be facilitated by lying down. In this observational study,119 lipedema patients were presented, the observations from the first publication from 1940 being confirmed.

Only 1 year later, Hines published another article on lipedema with the title "Lipedema and physiologic edema." Here, he continues to speak of adipose tissue proliferation and water accumulation in lipedema. What was new was the exclusion of the feet region in the description of fatty deposits or edema. The absence of edema in the feet was explained by tight-fitting shoes that could have prevented it.

These three studies were therefore the "birth" of lipedema as a disease and are still quoted today. Many of the facts described here have retained their validity, but there are also some aspects that we now see differently. One example of this is the term "progressive" disease, which we discuss in more detail in Sect. 1.5.

▶   Cited facts about lipedema often come from rather older studies and do not meet current scientific standards.

Let's get to one of the biggest misconceptions about lipedema:
"Lipedema is a condition associated with lymphedema."
This statement is wrong and has been outdated for a long time. Regrettably, however, this has yet to be understood by those affected, by the press and a significant number of scientific papers.

Rare cases in which there a combination of lipedema and lymphedema can be diagnosed clinically make the exception to this claim. Moreover, the outdated disease name suggests that it is edema, which in the true sense, it is not but rather pathologically distributed fat tissue.

▶   The first three publications on lipedema are:
▶   Allen EV, Hines EA (1940) Lipedema of the legs: a syndrome characterized by fat legs and orthostatic edema. Proc Staff Meet Mayo Clin. 15: 184–187.
▶   Wold LE, Hines EA Jr., Allen EV (1951) Lipedema of the legs; a syndrome characterized by fat legs and edema. Ann Intern Med 34(5): 1243–1250.
▶   Hines EA Jr. (1952) Lipedema and "Physiologic" Edema. Proc Staff Meet Mayo Clin 27(1): 7–9.
▶   Lipedema is a real disease that must be taken seriously.

1.2   Causes and Emergence

In this section, among other things, we want to go on causal research and talk about the pathophysiology of lipedema. We will not only discuss our own knowledge but also go into those facts that are unfortunately far too often sold as truths. You can expect an exciting potpourri of scientifically proven facts, hypotheses, suppositions, half-truths as well as insights gained from observations.

The term "pathophysiology" is composed of two terms. The word "pathology" comes from the ancient Greek πάθος, páthos, meaning "disease," and λόγος, lógos, the doctrine. Pathology, then, means the doctrine of disease, the "doctrine of afflictions." The word physiology is also composed of two words and comes from the ancient Greek: φύσις, phýsis, 'nature' and λόγος, lógos, 'doctrine'. Physiology is consequently the study of what is normal or healthy. Pathophysiology thus describes which functional mechanisms lead to pathological changes and how the sick body functions.

Before we turn to the pathophysiology, we must briefly discuss the disease triggering factors. To date, the trigger mechanism for a fat distribution disorder is unknown. Also, why lipohypertrophy that it can be an inherited condition (the literature speaks of an accumulation of up to 60% in first-degree relatives). In addition, there are factors such as hormonal balance and lifestyle. But one thing is certain: lipedema takes place in or around the adipose tissue. That is why we are taking a closer look at the adipose tissue.

▶   Triggers of lipohypertrophy and lipedema are unknown.

1.2.1   Adipose Tissue

When talking about adipose tissue, we distinguish between "storage fat" and "constitutional" fat. We find the constitutional fat mainly in the area of organs such as the kidney, but also in our extremities, such as the hands and feet. In the area of the heel, it serves, among other things, to absorb shocks when walking, thus the fat having here a purely mechanical function. The storage fat is the classic subcutaneous adipose tissue, which acts as an energy storage reserve and "cold insulation" or insulator.

Types
We distinguish a total of three types of adipose tissue: white, beige, and brown adipose tissue (Fig. 1.2). In the context of lipedema, only the white adipose tissue, which has the function of storage or depot fat, is of interest to us.

However, before we take a closer look at white adipose tissue, for the sake of completeness we will briefly discuss the other two forms.

Until 2009, it was assumed that brown adipose tissue was only present in babies. However, a study showed that adults also have a proportion—albeit very small—of brown fat. Brown fat has the property that it can generate heat. This occurs in the so-called mitochondria, which work like small power plants within the cells. This

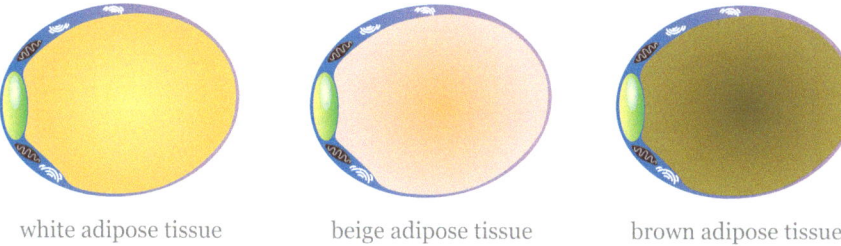

white adipose tissue   beige adipose tissue   brown adipose tissue

Fig. 1.2 White, beige, and brown adipose tissue

form of adipose tissue is very common in the animal kingdom, especially in animals that hibernate so it will help them to quickly raise their body temperature as soon as they wake up. Adults, on the other hand, have only limited brown fat depots.

Beige adipose tissue is found sporadically between the white adipose tissue. The function is not conclusively clarified; however, heat production is also discussed.

Let us now turn to the white adipose tissue. We find this as subcutaneous adipose tissue all over the body and thus also in the regions where lipedema takes place.

The subcutaneous fat tissue, where lipedema takes place, consists of white adipose tissue.

Adipose tissue is a form of connective tissue and consists, among other things, of fat cells, the so-called adipocytes. One can imagine adipose tissue as a sponge in which the "holes" are filled with adipocytes. The adipocytes are surrounded by many other different cells, scaffolding fibers and blood vessels and are combined within the surrounding tissue into small conglomerates, so-called lobules. Also located in the adipocyte environment are the progenitor cells of the adult adipocyte, which we will look at in more detail later in this section.

Depending on the body region, the subcutaneous fat tissue is structured differently. The total layer of subcutaneous fat tissue is divided into two compartments by a fat fascia (connective tissue plate): superficial and deep. The superficial compartment contains predominantly finer fat cells, while the deep compartment contains larger fat cells or fat conglomerates, each in proportion to the respective region. This means that, for example, the conglomerates of the deep fat layer on the buttocks are much larger than those on the forearm. In Fig. 1.3, we see an example of such a structure.

The white adipose tissue has different functions. In addition to its function as a metabolic organ, it mainly acts as a storage or depot fat. In addition, it can act as insulating fat to protect against heat loss and as a buffer zone as well as a protective layer in the form of building fat (kidney-bearing fat, sole of foot, eye).

▶   The largest proportion of white adipose tissue is found in the subcutaneous adipose tissue.

Structure and Function
Similar to the way human skin acts as a barrier to the environment, a fat cell (adipocyte) is separated from the environment by a cell membrane (cell wall).

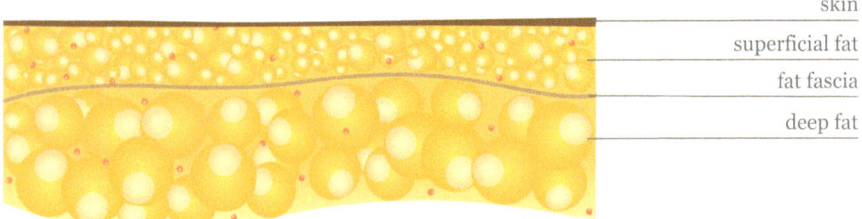

skin
superficial fat
fat fascia
deep fat

Fig. 1.3 Adipose tissue buildup in the subcutaneous fat tissue

This cell wall contains a number of different interfaces to which messenger substances can dock and trigger cell actions. We call these interface receptors. Examples are estrogen, insulin, and adrenaline receptors. In lipedema, receptors seem to play a central role. Therefore, we will go into this topic again in more detail in Sect. 1.2.3.

The fat cell, like any cell, has a "basic equipment," that is, a typical cell structure with a nucleus, where the genetic information (DNA) is located, with its energy providing mitochondrial apparatus and so on. Within the fat cell are the cell organelles, surrounded by the cytoplasm with the basic water-based structure of the cell, the cytosol. These are responsible for different functions of the cell.

The special feature of each white fat cell is its function of storing fat. The fat inside the cell is not limited by any wall or similar. The so-called lipid droplet (the fat content in the fat cell) is delimited in the cell only by a light-colored fringe (delimiting vimentin filaments) visible under the microscope. Depending on whether one or more fat droplets are found in the fat cell, we distinguish univacuolar (one fat droplet) from multivacuolar fat (several fat droplets) whereas white adipose tissue is predominantly univacuolar fat.

In Fig. 1.4 we show an example of a univacuolar fat cell with a typical, voluminous lipid droplet accounting for about 95% of the cell volume, pushing the nucleus to the cell membrane forming a so-called signet ring structure of the cell nucleus.

The energy balance of our body is subject to a constant dynamic. We distinguish between an anabolic and a catabolic phase. During the anabolic phase, the body's own energy storage components are built up under a certain energy consumption. For fat cells, this means that the lipid droplet is built up as a fat store in an anabolic phase and broken down accordingly in a catabolic phase.

A buildup and storage of fatty acids in a fat cell is only possible when there is an energetic surplus. The storage of energy in fat form is only possible through two mechanisms:

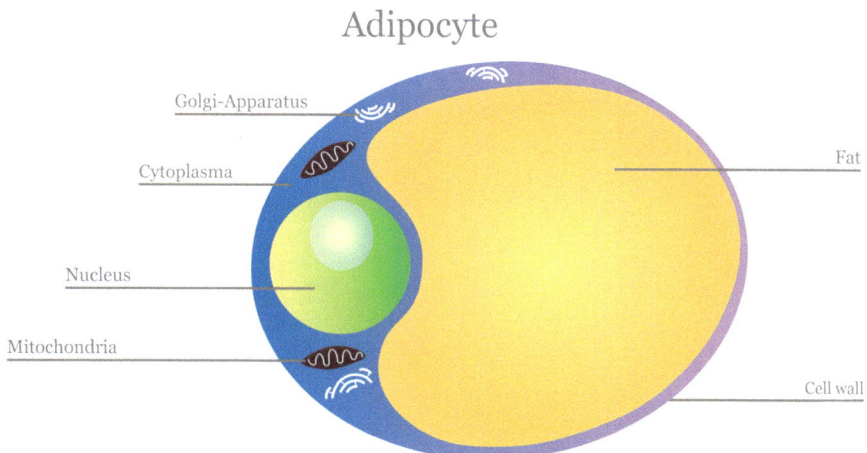

Fig. 1.4 Univacular fat cell with typical giant lipid droplet

1. absorption and storage of fats via food intake or,
2. body's own production of fatty acids, for example, by carbohydrates, a process is also known as fatty acid synthesis.

The breakdown of fatty acids and the resulting energy is referred to as lipolysis. The buildup and breakdown of fat are hormonally controlled, the hormones insulin and adrenaline play being the key players in this process.

Did you know that a fat cell has a limited lifespan and is subject to a life cycle? Fat cells are continuously built up and broken down by the body. An adult adipocyte grows from a fat precursor cell, a so-called preadipocyte, which in turn grows from a connective tissue precursor cell. You are probably wondering now how a fat cell knows that it is to become a fat cell? For the differentiation or development of such a fat cell, several intricate messenger compounds and processes are required. Explained simply, there is something like a program that is played leading to the production of all the necessary messengers so that the precursor cells understand that they need to turn into a fat cell. When the life of the fat cell is over, it dies and is degraded. A new fat cell develops in its place (Fig. 1.5).

If we take another look at the structure of adipose tissue, we have to imagine a convolute of fat cells, blood vessels, and other connective tissue cells. The so-called precursor cells (stem cells) are attached to the small blood vessels, from which new, young fat cells can develop by means of appropriate signals. In the process, they take up appropriate triglycerides (fatty acids) from the blood, through which they build up your fat droplet.

Body fat tissue can expand from 2–3% to over 60–70% of the body volume. A normal weight man has a fat tissue percentage of about 10–20%, a woman about 15–25%.

In childhood and adolescence, there is an increase in the absolute number of fat cells, but in adulthood, their numbers remain under physiological conditions

Life cycle of fat cell

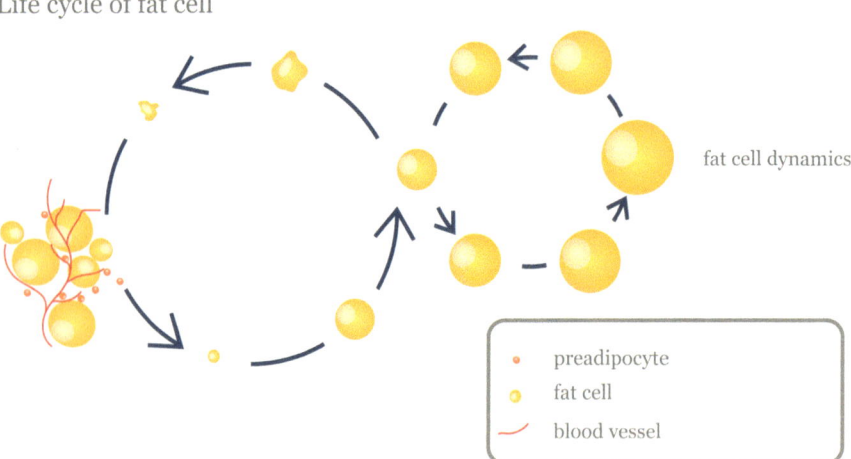

fat cell dynamics

- preadipocyte
- fat cell
- blood vessel

Fig. 1.5 The picture shows the theoretical life cycle of a fat cell

unchanged. Weight gain will lead to an increase in the size of the existing fat cells whereas, in the case of weight loss, the opposite happens. In these cases, we speak of hyperplasia and hypertrophy of fat cells. Hyperplasia stands for the proliferation of fat cells (an increase of their absolute numbers) and hypertrophy stands for a pure increase in the volume of each individual fat cell.

▷ The number of adult fat cells increases until puberty without significant change afterwards. What can still change in adulthood is the volume of the individual fat cells.

Even after massive weight loss following bariatric surgery, it was shown that the absolute fat cell count did not change significantly.

About 8.4% of all fat cells renew themselves each year. It is assumed that each fat cell has a lifespan of about 1 year. In total, a normal average person with 13.5 kg of adipose tissue has about 40 billion fat cells.

A fat cell can store a maximum of 1 μg of fat (= 1 millionth of a gram = 10 − 6 g). 1 g of fat has about 7 calories.

▷ 1 kg of fat tissue has 7000 calories. If you wanted to lose 1 kg of fat in a week, you would therefore have to save 1000 calories a day (at constant body weight).

Due to our physical storage and depot fat, humans are able to go several days without food.

▷ One cubic centimeter of fat (equivalent to the volume of 1 mL of water) weighs 0.94 g. 1 L of fat is therefore equivalent to 940 g.

In humans, there are different types of fat storage depending on gender. We speak of a gender-typical fat distribution, in a variable range that is genetically determined (Fig. 1.6).

A study on the structure of adipose tissue of lipedema patients as compared to and healthy individuals (both groups were of normal weight), revealed enlarged fat cells in the lipedema group.

1.2.2 Science in Detail

For the understanding and treatment of disease, science is the measure of all things. For this reason, we need to look at the scientific data on lipedema to delve further into the topic of pathophysiology. However, not all science is the same. We distinguish different qualities of scientific papers. The measure of the quality of a scientific paper is measured by a level of evidence. A good paper has a high degree of evidence and thus also a high content of truth of its statements. The basis of a good paper starts in the planning phase with the basic framework, the study design. If the

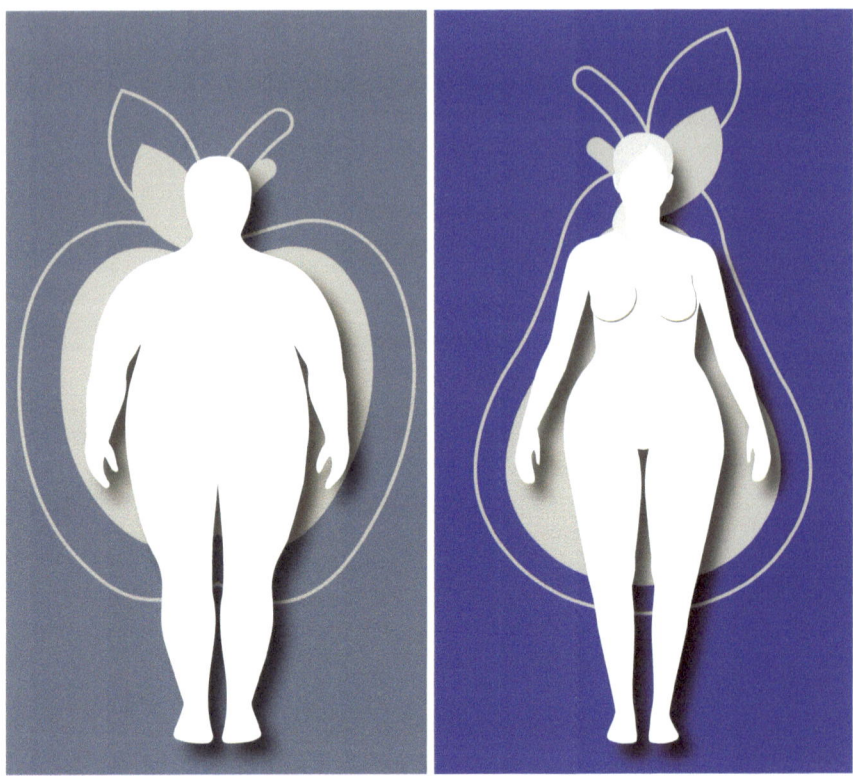

Fig. 1.6 Gender-typical fat distribution in men (apple type) and women (pear type)

design of the study is not well planned, no meaningful result will emerge at the end of the work.

Such examples are observational studies that focus mainly on one single question and not on a certain intervention (e.g., how pain perception changes in lipedema patients after surgery) aimed to improve outcomes. Thus, the overall results of such a study, regardless of being retrospective or prospective remain of limited relevance for the reader. It is why, one should choose carefully the information sources, be aware of the relevance of each information, and not believe in everything that's written.

Purely scientifically, we do not know much about lipedema. The scientific papers that exist on lipedema are rather poor in terms of scientific quality. Most of the studies we found are purely descriptive or observational, underpinned by conclusions and references of other equally poor studies. Experimental studies on lipedema are extremely rare to find. The few studies that do exist use questionable study designs, small numbers of cases, or fail to show statistically significant results.

Anyone who still has doubts about this shocking reality should independently perform the same search on the subject lipedema. As such, affirmations like: "Lipedema is curable" or "The diseased fat cells store water instead of fat" appearing either on websites or other media, are grossly negligent and without any scientific fundament. Updating a patient about the actual stand of knowledge in lipedema is a tedious but mandatory step before initiating the talk on possible treatment options. As a consequence, many patients leave after the first consultation dissatisfied, because of being confronted with an uncomfortable truth. This fact is also frustrating for the physician, his efforts to provide such information in a reasonable way to his patients resemble at times a battle against windmills.

Let us first look at the general data situation. If we search for the term "lipedema" in one of the largest scientific portals (PubMed), we currently (01/2020) find a total of 197 literature hits, although this number says nothing about the really correct hit rate on the topic and certainly nothing about the quality of the studies. If we search for the term "lymphedema," there are 15,203 hits.

It is claimed that up to every tenth woman suffers from lipedema. We have similar disease figures with breast cancer. Although breast cancer, which can have fatal consequences, is not comparable to lipedema, the 399,260 hits when entering "breast cancer" in the search mask demonstrate how underrepresented lipedema is in the scientific literature. This is also clear in the case of lymphedema, which occurs much less frequently than lipedema, but has many times more hits.

Of the 197 hits in the literature about lipedema, we believe that about 80% have major relevance issues. The remaining 20% include good studies in terms of structure and design, but none could be found in which the following questions are clearly answered:

1. How is the disease triggered?
2. What is the mechanism of the disease?
3. How can lipedema be diagnosed with certainty?
4. How can the disease be cured?

Consequently, we are largely dealing with observations and assertions in these studies. Unfortunately, and this is currently a problem, many statements from these studies have managed to be recognized as truths and facts. To our regret, this recognition has occurred not only among patients and their families but also among many physicians who propagate these findings instead of questioning them. Almost every patient referred to us with the diagnosis of lipedema will say "I have lipedema and water in my legs." This statement is more than questionable since lipedema primarily has nothing to do with water retention. As already described in Sect. 1.2.1, a fat cell consists largely of lipids and only to a small extent of water, which is present in the form of the cytosol. There are rare exceptions, which we will discuss in more detail in Sect. 1.3.

An interesting phenomenon: Germany is at the forefront of scientific publications on lipedema. At this point, however, we are only looking at the absolute number of publications and not the quality. In addition, Germany is also a pioneer in scientifically unfounded statements on this topic.

Guidelines for diseases are often published by professional societies or an association of professional societies. This is also the case with lipedema. These guidelines are available to all on the Internet and, like studies, are divided into different quality classes. The lipedema guideline is a so-called S1 guideline with only a "recommendation" character. Here, too, there is a lack of scientific impact because the guideline reflects the opinions of various experts. There are no objective criteria that make one an expert or not. Just as we have not been tested as experts, but consider ourselves to be.

▶   Anyone can download the current guidelines for the treatment of lipedema from the AWMF website at https://www.awmf.org/

1.2.3   Hormone Activity of the Adipose Tissue

The hormonal activity of the adipose tissue is an often underestimated aspect of lipedema. Adipose tissue has long since ceased to be regarded as an inactive, inert tissue, being much more than a mere "fat store." It is an active and also endocrine organ. The metabolism of adipose tissue affects the entire body. Adipose tissue is capable of synthesizing and releasing hormones but is also sensitive to hormones such as estrogen and insulin.

Since the onset of lipedema often coincides with the onset of a hormonal change phase, an estrogen-regulated disorder is assumed. Whether this is inherited polygenetically (i.e., a change resulting from several gene changes) or monogenetically is still a subject of research. Based on our clinical observation and the stories of the affected persons, a hormonal connection is also comprehensible from our point of view.

Estrogen
We have already talked about the life cycle as well as the metabolism of fat cells. Another theory, which has been researched with scientifically sound and comprehensible foundations, focuses precisely on this metabolism and the control of the fat cell by estrogens. Estrogens are recognized by two different receptors of the fat cell. We distinguish the estrogen receptor α (alpha) from the estrogen receptor β (beta). Both receptors trigger different metabolic mechanisms in the fat cell. At the same time, these receptors are also found on many other tissue cells; we will focus here and now on the fat cell. In the schematic representation, we have omitted other receptors for simplicity (Fig. 1.7).

Fig. 1.7 Schematic representation of estrogen receptors on a fat cell

Fat Cell Estrogen Receptor

Estrogen Receptor (α) ❚

Estrogen Receptor (β) ❚

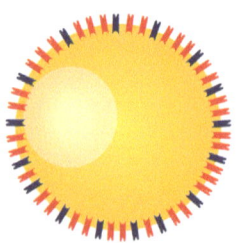

The α-receptor is significantly responsible for energy balance (buildup and breakdown of fat volume), the inflammatory response in adipose tissue and fibrosis.

▶   Fibrosis is a pathological proliferation of connective tissue that results from increased collagen synthesis. Fibrosed connective tissue is hardened and functionless. If, for example, lung tissue turns fibrotic, this part is no longer available for gas exchange.

If the estrogen concentration is reduced (e.g., postmenopausally), abdominal obesity develops with an increased risk of metabolic syndrome. This development can be counteracted, for example, by estrogen replacement therapy.

In addition to the concentration of estrogen in the bloodstream, an incorrect (pathological) distribution pattern of α- and β-estrogen receptors on fat cells can program "fat gain" or "fat loss" (Fig. 1.8).

The α-estrogen receptor mostly triggers positive metabolic processes. By this, we mean an improvement in insulin sensitivity and glucose tolerance. The receptor counteracts fat accumulation, which is why it is attributed a weight-reducing property. Overall, its triggered metabolic cascades lead to a normalization of fat and sugar balance.

To explain: Each fat cell carries an individual number of α- and β-estrogen receptors. Their distribution determines how a fat cell responds to caloric excess (Fig. 1.9). Many of these conclusions have emerged from animal studies. If these theories apply to humans, then this theory would be a reasonable explanation of why lipedema develops in some women and not in others. Indeed, if the α-receptor were increased and the β-receptor decreased on a fat cell, adipose tissue would be degraded; the other way around, the fat gain would occur.

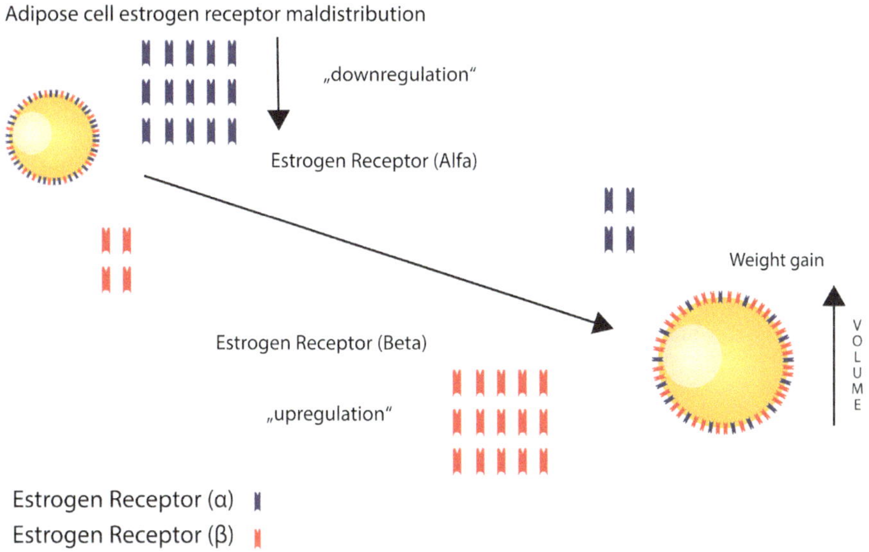

Adipose cell estrogen receptor maldistribution

Fig. 1.8 Schematic maldistribution of estrogen receptors that can lead to weight gain

Development of Lipedema

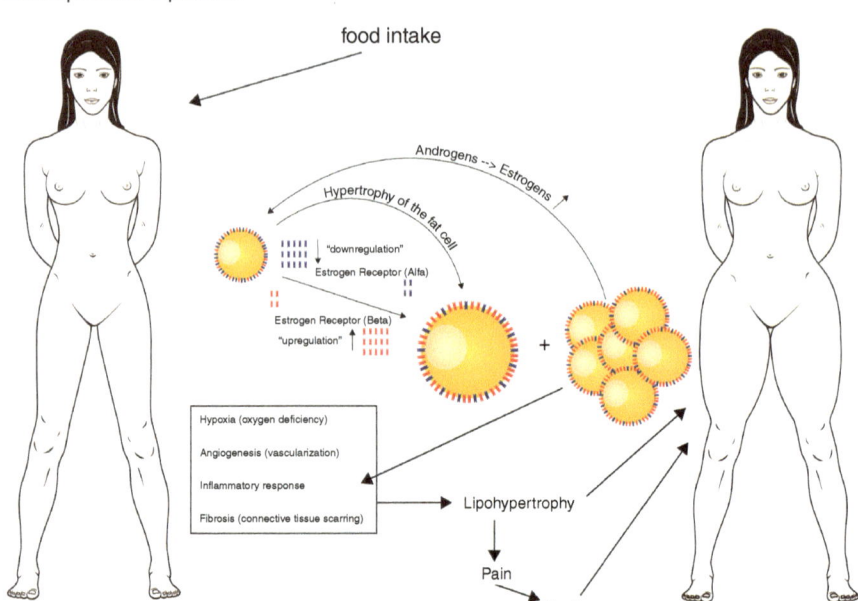

Fig. 1.9 Illustration of lipedema development

> ▶ Adipose tissue is hormone-active and hormone-sensitive. In lipedema, a
>   maldistribution of estrogen receptors in the area of the affected regions
>   is assumed.

In addition, altered estrogen receptor patterns in the brain are discussed as causative for impaired appetite.

Estrogen and Progesterone

The counterpart of estrogen is progesterone. Progesterone is a so-called corpus
luteum hormone and the most important representative of the progestins, which—as
the name suggests—are produced in the corpus luteum of the ovaries. The balance
between progesterone and estrogen is of enormous importance for our body. If there
is a disbalance, important body functions such as weight regulation become
unbalanced.

Since estrogen production in adipose tissue occurs through the conversion of
androgens (male sex hormones) into estrogen, too much adipose tissue leads to
estrogen overproduction. This acts on the own estrogen receptors and at the same
time causes a further imbalance to progesterone.

If the estrogen level is permanently elevated compared to the progesterone level
due to a lot of existing adipose tissue, overeating, or due to an underproduction of
progesterone in the ovaries, there will be a continuous weight gain. The situation is
similar during menopause. Although there is a lack of estrogen, at the same time

hardly any progesterone is produced due to the absence of ovulation, so that there is also a disbalance.

▶   When there is an excess of estrogen, we speak of estrogen dominance.
▶   In women over 40, there is additional energy saving due to a failure of ovulation. If egg production is reduced or comes to a complete standstill, the body saves up to 300 kcal a day 1 week before the period.

Insulin

Insulin is also an important hormone for fat metabolism. But what is insulin and what does it do exactly? Insulin is a hormone that is produced and released by the pancreas. A release of insulin occurs with food intake which in turn will regulate the sugars extracted from food to can be taken from the bloodstream into our body cells.

It works according to the lock-and-key principle. Insulin is the key that docks with a receptor on the cell surface and can then introduce sugar molecules into the cell.

If obesity is present, this can lead to so-called insulin resistance. This means that the insulin signal no longer has its intended effect. In principle, more and more insulin release leads to overstimulation of the receptors. The overstimulation causes the insulin receptors to down-regulate ("down-regulate"). As a result, the cells can no longer respond adequately to insulin secretion. The pancreas in turn tries to compensate for this by overproducing insulin, which can be up to 15 times the original amount of insulin. Eventually, however, the pancreas gives up and stops producing insulin. The result is a chronically elevated blood glucose level, type II diabetes.

▶   The consequence of insulin resistance is the so-called "diabetes" = diabetes type II.

The result of insulin resistance is further weight gain through the following mechanisms: no longer enough glucose reaches the cells because the insulin key can no longer open the gate for sugar (glucose). In the brain, too, insulin can induce appetite suppression, which does not occur when there is resistance. Thus, there is a lack of central inhibition of appetite. This can cause you to get a strong craving for sugary foods and then logically follow that, supporting the vicious cycle. Researchers made an interesting discovery in this area. They found that the amount of belly fat increases in particular the risk of insulin resistance by up to 80%. In comparison, fat in other parts of the body only increases the risk of this by 50–60%.

Excessive blood glucose levels are extremely harmful to the body in the long term. Particularly susceptible to "hyperglycemia" are the small and smallest blood vessels, which undergo pathological changes. This results in circulatory disorders, for example, in the kidneys and the eye, but also in vascular changes in large blood vessels, such as those in the legs (PAD—peripheral arterial occlusive disease) which will, in turn, increase the risk of heart disease and stroke.

- ▶ If the symptoms occur
- ▶ elevated blood glucose level,
- ▶ Severe overweight.
- ▶ High blood pressure and.
- ▶ Lipid metabolism disorders.
- ▶ together, we speak of a "metabolic syndrome."

As suspected, the known risk factors for developing diabetes are obesity due to overeating, heredity, stress, and lack of exercise. Generally speaking, when a body is "fed" glucose, it causes a shift in metabolism. Fat breakdown is slowed down and the synthesis of new fat is pushed.

Leptin

Another hormone produced by fat cells is leptin. In healthy people, leptin reduces appetite. Unfortunately, this is not the case in people with an increased amount of fat. Although leptin levels are higher than in normal-weight individuals due to the mass of adipose tissue, the brains of obese people respond to leptin more poorly than those of healthy individuals. We call this condition, analogous to insulin, leptin resistance. Why the brain fails to reach the full leptin message is still a subject of research. Due to leptin resistance, a feeling of satiety is often not achieved despite sumptuous meals, and the appetite remains. This leads to an unstoppable urge to eat, which accelerates the vicious circle.

Ghrelin

Ghrelin is the hunger hormone par excellence, a growth hormone that is produced predominantly in the stomach, but also to a small extent in the pancreas. Via the bloodstream, it reaches our central mainboard (brain) and interacts with the hunger center and the pineal gland. Ghrelin stimulates the pineal gland to secrete the growth hormone somatotropin. A deficiency of somatotropin in an adult is associated with obesity, decreased life expectancy, reduced muscle mass, and decreased bone density. Before food intake and during periods of fasting, serum ghrelin levels in the blood increase. Normally, food intake results in suppression of ghrelin release. Curiously, one would think otherwise low ghrelin secretion occurs in obesity, however, this is still under investigation, one possible theory suggests that obese people are more sensitive to the hormone ghrelin.

- ▶ It is reasonable to assume that hormonal changes can trigger or aggravate lipedema.

Basically, we must note that lipedema is often associated with obesity and obesity is often associated with lipedema.

- ▶ Adipose tissue is very hormone-active.

The adipose tissue in lipedema is normal adipose tissue in terms of its rough structure. However, it is still special, because due to altered receptors on the fat cell surface (still a subject of research), adipose tissue in lipedema behaves differently than "normal" adipose tissue—and this is undisputed.

1.2.4 Lipohypertrophy

A widely accepted theory on the development of lipedema is that of "lipohypertrophy." From our point of view, this is a theory that makes sense in many patients but at the same time disregards a number of patients with atypical lipedema (Fig. 1.10). Affected persons with atypical lipedema often have severe pain and above-average suffering.

The theory of "lipohypertrophy" states the following: The basic prerequisite for lipedema to develop is the prior presence of lipohypertrophy. Lipohypertrophy is a multifactorial fat distribution disorder of the buttocks, hips, legs, and/or arms. Only one or several different regions may be affected. Heredity plays a central role in the development of lipohypertrophy, as do environmental influences, diet, and lifestyle habits. The approach with the estrogen receptor distribution disorder is particularly

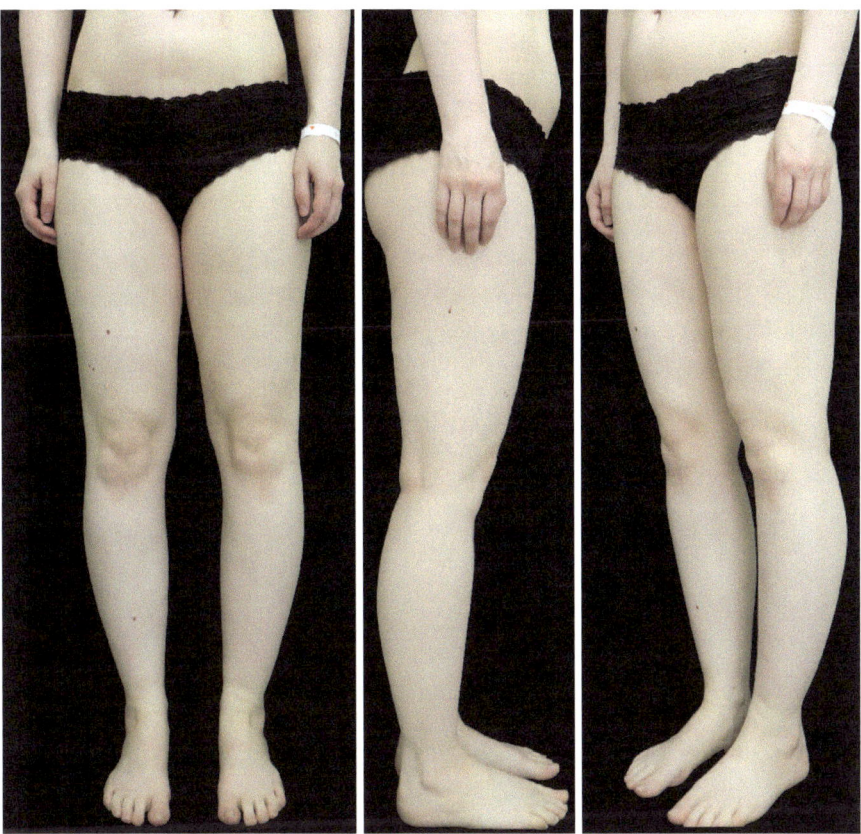

Fig. 1.10 A lipedema of an affected person not recognizable at first sight

comprehensible in lipohypertrophy. Lipohypertrophy is by definition always painless.

▶ Fat distribution disorder (lipohypertrophy) is multifactorial; especially the hereditary component seems to play a major role. Lipohypertrophy is not accompanied by pain.

Lipohypertrophy varies greatly from individual to individual and, in extreme cases, can be such that the waist is extremely slender and the legs very voluminous (Fig. 1.11). From a purely external point of view, lipohypertrophy cannot be easily distinguished from lipedema.

Figure 1.12 shows a typical clinical picture of lipohypertrophy.

Lipedema then develops from this lipohypertrophy. Externally, it can look absolutely identical, but as soon as pain is added as a leading symptom to lipohypertrophy, we speak of lipedema. In this theory, therefore, lipedema does not develop directly, but develops out of lipohypertrophy, which by definition is painless.

At the other extreme are very slim women who have a barely visible fat distribution disorder. Many outsiders, who are not familiar with the subject, wrongly condemn these women. Often these women search for a perceived eternity until the correct diagnosis is made.

We refer to the lipedema in these women as "atypical lipedema," since visible lipohypertrophy is only indicated or completely absent, but the typical pain due to the adipose tissue is still present.

▶ A fat distribution disorder simply means a disturbed distribution of fat tissue on the body and, by definition, is not associated with pain.

What is the difference between lipohypertrophy and lipedema? The most important distinguishing feature is the symptomatology in terms of pain.

The lady in the picture may have lipohypertrophy or she may have lipedema. Typically, these findings are often pure lipohypertrophy without pain. In this case (Fig. 1.13), the affected person stated pain, which by definition makes it lipedema.

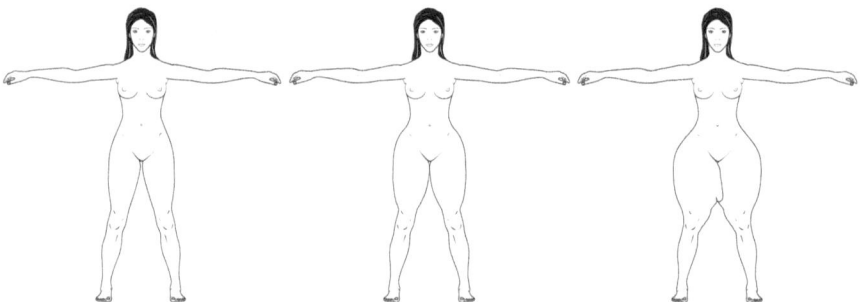

Fig. 1.11 Exemplary manifestation of lipohypertrophy

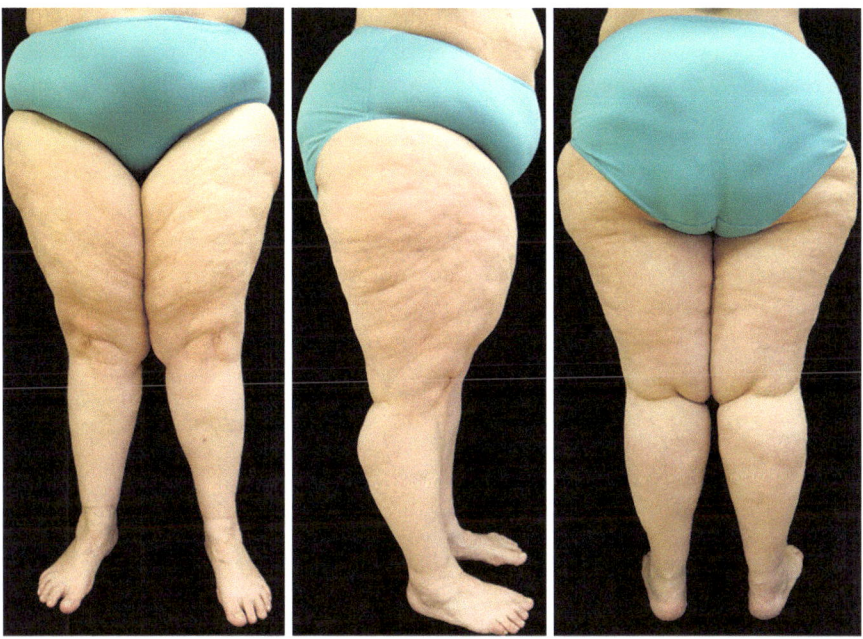

Fig. 1.12 Clinical example of lipohypertrophy

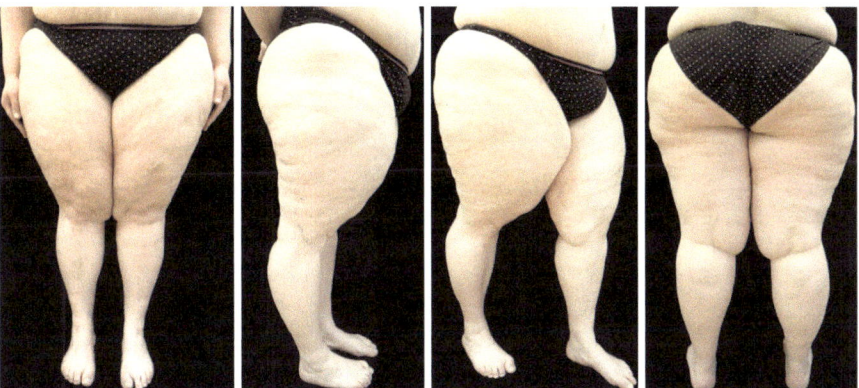

Fig. 1.13 Lipohypertrophy or lipedema?

▶ If someone suffers from a disproportion in favor of buttocks, hips, legs, and/or arms without pain, then it is per se a "lipohypertrophy," that is, a pure fat distribution disorder.

▶ If the same person has complaints in the sense of pressure, touch, rest or stress pain, then we call this condition "lipedema."

The risk that initially painless lipohypertrophy will develop into painful lipedema increases with the further development of the disproportion, that is, a further increase in fat tissue. The further increase can have different causes, for example, a further hormonal change with downstream metabolic changes or also a pure calorie surplus due to malnutrition can be responsible for it. We will discuss why the pain develops in Sect. 1.4.

Regardless of whether or not someone suffers from a genetic predisposition to a fat distribution disorder, hormonal transition phases are often associated with weight gain. Perhaps you have experienced it yourself. You are like many women in whom pregnancy and often the onset of menopause lead to an increase in body weight. In the case of a fat distribution disorder, however, the fat tissue is then distributed differently. Thus, simply a further continuous weight gain can also lead to a further expression of the disproportion and the lipohypertrophy can turn into a painful lipedema.

In Fig. 1.14, we want to show you the range of different manifestations of lipedema.

In each affected person, lipohypertrophy is objectively present whether lipedema can only be determined by including the subjective "pain."

Very often we see that in the internet portals and literature a certain type of lipedema is described as "typical lipedema." We consider such a description to be misleading. Considering the wide range of different manifestations of lipedema, it is difficult to speak of "a typical lipedema" in our view. In fact, all women in the pictures shown in Fig. 1.14 complained about "pain" and thus suffer from lipedema by definition.

Almost all theories agree that in lipedema individual fat cells increase. Some experts from different fields—and we do not share their opinion—postulate that there is also an increase in the total number of fat cells. Advocates of this theory also argue that the preliminary stage of lipedema should not be called "lipohypertrophy." Rather, the preliminary stage of lipedema should be referred to as "latency stage lipedema syndrome" (i.e., not yet erupted). We consider this view to be rather absurd since substantial scientifical evidence exists on the fact that there is no, and if only very subordinate, increase in the absolute number of fat cells in lipedema.

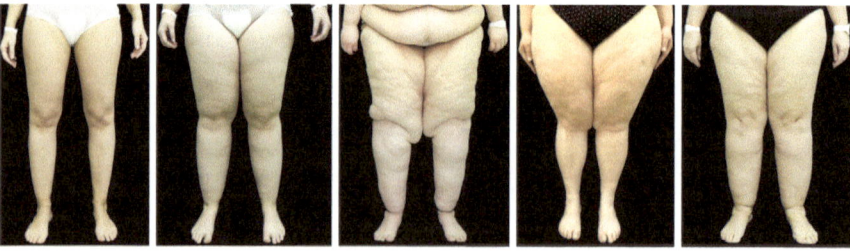

Fig. 1.14 Different manifestations of lipedema

▶   If a cell (e.g., fat cell) increases in volume, we speak in the technical jargon of "hypertrophy." If there is an increase in the absolute number of cells, we speak of "hyperplasia."

1.2.5   Theory of Microvascular Disruption and Lymphatic Interaction

To understand the development of lipedema, two main theories must be considered: one is the theory of microvascular dysfunction, the other is the theory of lymphatic interaction.

In microvascular disorders, it is assumed that an increase in fat cell volume causes an undersupply of oxygen to the tissue. The oxygen deficiency is a stimulus for new blood vessel formation because the body wants to counteract the deficiency with new vessel sprouting. This results in malformed capillaries, which should explain the tendency to hematoma.

The theory of lymphatic interaction states that the lymphatic and capillary vascular systems act incorrectly, resulting in the formation of edema. Local messengers and degradation products produced by metabolic processes interact with the local fat cells, resulting in a slow change of the tissue. The result is hypertrophy (enlargement) of the fat cell and fibrosis (proliferation and hardening due to increased collagen synthesis) of the connective tissue. Likewise, a chronic, subliminal inflammatory reaction of the tissue is said to play a role, which is mainly responsible for fibrosis.

We can confirm from our clinical observation that fibrosis does indeed occur (Fig. 1.15). During liposuction procedures, we see clear differences in tissue quality between patients or even body areas and whether liposuction is "easy" or rather "laborious" during the performance.

If we look at pure lymphedema, we often see an increase in subcutaneous fat tissue here as well, which would argue in favor of this theory.

1.2.6   Uncontrolled Fat Tissue Proliferation

We often read and hear that the adipose tissue in lipedema would "proliferate." The adipose tissue is said to virtually take on a life of its own and inexorably increase in volume, no matter what. For this book, we looked for scientific evidence of this uncontrolled growth and proliferation of adipose tissue but found no solid proof.

There is not even a rudimentary basis of argumentation for this. In medicine, we are only familiar with uncontrolled growth in tumor tissue (benign or malignant tissue proliferation). In lipedema, however, we are not dealing with a tumor disease, but with storage of excess energy in the form of fat in fat cells. The peculiarity, in our opinion, is that in classic lipedema there is a fat distribution disorder, regardless of the possible causes, and therefore there is the well-known visual fat distribution disorder. An uncontrolled growth would be accompanied by consumption of the

Fig. 1.15 Clinical picture of lymphedema with malapposed lymphatic vessels on the left side

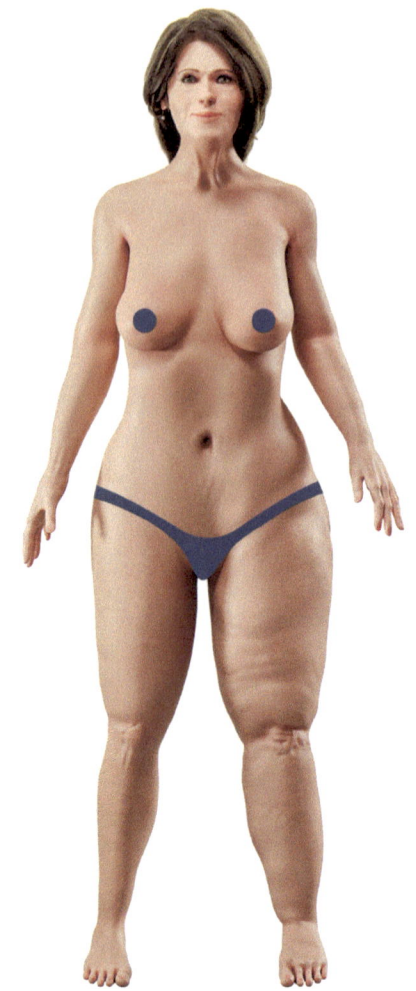

existing energy stores and not by a buildup of energy stores as in lipedema. We see this in the sad courses of advanced cancer, where the last reserves are drained from the body and it gradually undergoes degradation.

There is scientific work that has observed that sufferers with lipedema may continue to gain weight despite dieting and a calorie-deficient diet of around 10%. This is a very interesting statement that certainly requires further clarification.

▶   Adipose tissue in lipohypertrophy and or lipedema does not proliferate uncontrollably in the sense of becoming independent.

It is certainly quite comfortable to say that it is uncontrolled growth, especially when countless diet attempts have failed and weight gain continues to occur. It is not the fault of the patient, because there is a complex malfunctioning system underlying the weight gain. When this has been understood, therapy can be successful.

1.3 The Edema

Let us now turn to the central point of discussion, the edema in lipedema. Colleagues, therapists and industry representatives still say today: "In lipedema, there is edema." Some claim this out of ignorance, others for monetary reasons because there is whole machinery behind the care of lipedema sufferers.

But what actually is edema, how does it develop, and how can we detect it? Colloquially, edema is often referred to as water retention. By definition, edemas are fluid deposits in the tissue. Many people first think of lymphedema. In brief, lymphedema is caused by a pathological change in the lymphatic system, for example, due to malpositioned lymphatic channels or surgically removed lymph nodes. This causes lymph to leak into the surrounding tissue, resulting in an increase in volume in the sense of lymphedema.

Depending on the disease, edema has different compositions. The main components of edema are water and proteins, in principle similar to blood plasma. If there is high protein content, we speak of protein-rich edema (so-called exudate), if there is a low protein concentration, we speak of protein-poor edema (so-called transudate).

Let's look again at lipedema and what we already know: Lipedema manifests itself in a circumscribed, symmetrically localized subcutaneous fat tissue proliferation, disturbed in distribution, in favor of the buttocks, hips, legs, and arms. In addition to this fat distribution disorder, edema may occur in rare cases; we then speak of lip-lymphedema or lipo-lymphedema.

The term "lipedema" has held up valiantly since it was first described in 1941. Unfortunately, the term was already unfavorable at that time because the first described was orthostatic edema (edema caused by gravity, usually in women due to prolonged standing or sitting). Perhaps you are familiar with this? This widespread edema also occurs in many healthy people, especially in summer. Like Hines, who initially described edema, I checked this out myself in the summer: I measured my leg circumferences right after I got up in the morning and at the end of a long consulting day. I am athletic, healthy, and fit. Yet, at the end of the day, I was able to measure a circumference increase of 3–5 mm on average. We are all subject to such minor variations throughout the day. Then there are the additional influencing factors such as weather, activity, and much more.

In many countries, knowledge about lipedema has already been consolidated to the extent that it is known that lipedema is not usually accompanied by edema requiring treatment. Therefore, we see the understanding of edema in lipedema as more of a national problem.

▶ In lipedema patients, there is usually no edema in the classical sense. Only very rarely are forms of combined lipedema or lipo-lymphedema seen.

Causes
Let's dive a little deeper into the subject of edema. If there is increased pressure in the venous circulatory system, fluid can be forced out of the bloodstream into the surrounding tissue. Most often we see this phenomenon in heart failure, so-called cardiac insufficiency, because the blood backs up in front of the heart, increasing the pressure in the venous part. Varicose veins in the legs may also be responsible for such increased pressure in the venous leg. Regardless of the causes, it is typically the legs that are affected by edema. The reason for this is gravity, which is followed by the fluid in the tissues and is thus deposited at the lowest point of the body.

Another cause of edema can be an altered colloid osmotic pressure in the blood. This sounds complicated however the facts are simply explained. To keep a certain amount of fluid in the blood vessels, the blood contains large protein molecules that attract the fluid to them. If the protein molecules are decreased, then the colloid osmotic pressure decreases and the proteins can no longer "hold" the fluid in the blood. The fluid migrates into the surrounding tissue, and edema develops. We often see edema in kidney diesease patients, for example, who lose a lot of protein in their urine. However, the lack of protein can also have another reason, for example, mal-nutrition, liver disease or metabolic disease.

Another possible cause of edema is vascular disease. This can result in increased permeability to fluids, which ultimately leads to fluid leakage into the surrounding connective tissue.

If a thrombosis (blockage of a blood vessel) develops or if there is a weakness of the venous valves in a leg vein, this also results in a backlog of venous blood with a corresponding increase in pressure in the system. The pressure forces fluid from the blood vessel system into the connective tissue.

Medications can also cause edema. Here, blood pressure medications and diuret-ics (water tablets) are at the top of the causative list. All of these edemas can undoubtedly be detected by ultrasound, MRI, or even other examinations (usually a simple indentation of the skin with the thumb is enough).

Theory of Increased Capillary Permeability
The most widespread theory of edema in lipedema is the theory of increased "capil-lary permeability." Lipedema is associated with, as the name suggests, increased permeability of the blood vessels (permeability) to proteins and water.

This happens at the level of the smallest vessels of the capillaries, a small but crucial section in our blood circulation (Fig. 1.16). Our blood circulation consists of arteries, veins and lymphatic vessels. Arteries carry oxygenated blood from the heart to the periphery, organs, brain, and all other tissues. At the capillary level, there is an exchange of oxygen, nutrients and waste products. This naturally results in some fluid transfer from the blood vessels and the capillary bed into the connec-tive tissue.

Fig. 1.16 Blood
circulation of the body

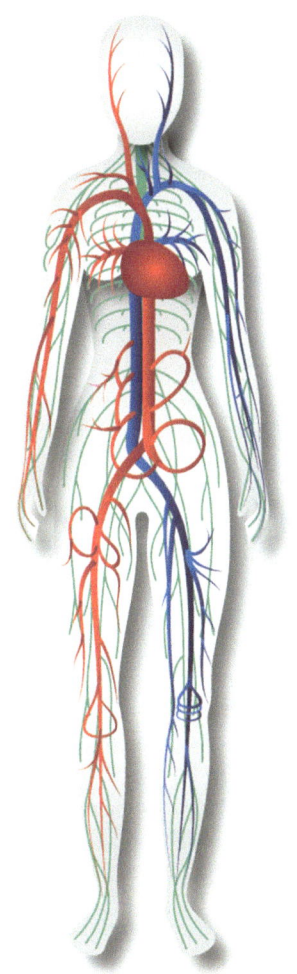

If there is increased capillary permeability for proteins (proteins) and water molecules, these pass into the connective tissue. Proteins are very large in relation to water molecules so that we speak here of macromolecules. They bind the water in the connective tissue and in this way cause manifest edema (Fig. 1.17).

Initially, the lymphatic system can still remove the increased tissue fluid and compensates for the situation. Many people speak here of a high-performance phase of the lymphatic system in the initial stage. However, after a longer period, this leads to an overload of the lymphatic system. This phase is also called the decompensation phase. In the further course, fibrosis of the lymphatic vessels occurs, resulting in a loss of inherent elasticity. This results in a further, progressive loss of function, and edema takes its course.

Change in capillary permeability

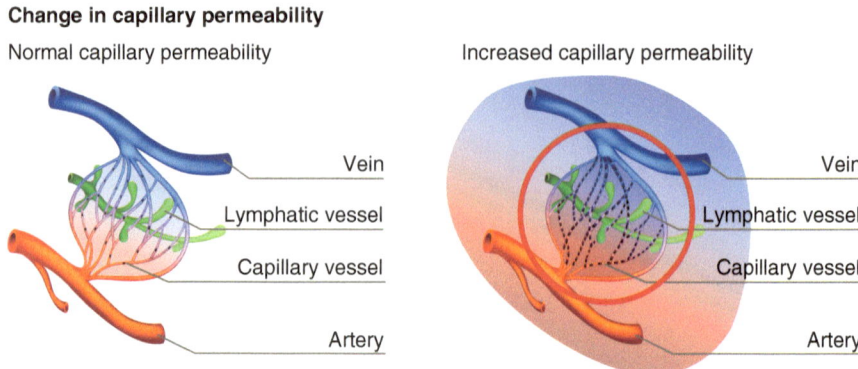

Normal capillary permeability   Increased capillary permeability

Vein   Vein

Lymphatic vessel   Lymphatic vessel

Capillary vessel   Capillary vessel

Artery   Artery

Fig. 1.17 Increased permeability of the capillary vessels

The capillaries not only become leaky to the proteins; it is suspected that they are then also more vulnerable than "healthy" capillaries. In this so-called microangiopathy, there is localized damage to the end-stream pathway with partial or complete loss of function of the smallest arteries (arterioles) and capillaries, so that they are injured more quickly and bruising can result.

The second explanation for the bruises we have just discussed is the theory with the lack of oxygen and the signal to the tissue: "We need more blood vessels." It should be noted that the new vessels suffer from capillary fragility and are more fragile than healthy vessels.

▶   Those affected by lipedema have a tendency to bruise (hematoma tendency).

Progression of lipedema results in further stretching of the lymphatic vessels and the formation of microaneurysms (vascular bulges). However, other studies contradict this theory. In our opinion, lipedema is not and does not remain a primary disease of the lymphatic system.

▶   We do not consider lipedema to be a primarily lymphatic disease.

Let's summarize the causes of edema in people suffering from lipedema:

As in healthy individuals who do not suffer from a painful fat distribution disorder, the most common type of edema is orthostatic edema (sagging of tissue fluid caused by the upright gait and gravity). The initial publication of lipedema also described edema in terms of "orthostatic edema," which occurs in response to position and weight-bearing. However, such edemas have nothing to do with lymphedema. Especially these edemas occur preferentially in the warm summer months.

Other causes can be the diseases described above. Of course, a combination of different causes is also possible.

Obesity-Associated Lymphedema
Let's now go into a little more detail about edema in overweight patients. There is a proven link between obesity and the development of leg edema. Approximately 20% of all German citizens are classified as obese. Among those suffering from edema, the proportion of obese people is significantly higher than in the normal population. Only up to 30% of edema patients have a normal BMI. Here, the question is certainly justified as to whether obesity or edema is present first since BMI inevitably increases with pronounced edema. We see obesity-associated lymphedema particularly in patients with a BMI above 40 kg/m².

Obesity-associated lymphedema, like lipedema, tends to be a diagnosis of exclusion. We typically observe the following circumstances:

– Lymphedema is not congenital and develops only in the second half of life.
– Lymphedema increases with weight.
– The feet are usually not affected, and Stemmer's sign (a diagnostic skin fold test after its first describer, Robert Stemmer, Sect. 1.9) need not be present because lymphedema tends to occur in the upper part of the lower extremity, that is, the buttocks, hips, upper and lower legs.
– We also see this form of edema in the area of fat aprons and the genital region.
– Skin changes are regularly observed in advanced stages.

The underlying pathological mechanism is represented by a circulatory disturbance of the lymphatic and venous systems due to the mass and deadweight of the adipose tissue and soft tissue excess. The vessels are "squeezed," which prevents further transport in the vascular system.

▶   If an increase in edema is observed along with weight gain, then these
     can often be positively influenced by weight loss.

We see edema in lipedema, especially in advanced stages. In these stages, there is usually also very pronounced obesity, so that it can be difficult to find the cause of the actual edema. Unfortunately, it is also not uncommon that water tablet abuse is practiced and thus edema is provoked.

In summary, so far, we can state the following reasons for the presence of lipo lymphedema:

– Presence of lipedema and lymphedema independently of each other.
– Obesity-associated lymphedema.
– Edema resulting from very advanced lipedema, even without obesity.

At first glance, it is often difficult to distinguish lipedema from lipo-lymphedema (Fig. 1.18). What do you think? Is it pure lipedema or lipo-lymphedema?

In this case, lipo-lymphedema is indeed present (Fig. 1.19). The lower legs and feet can be pressed in with a dent remaining for a long time as a result, which is indicative of lymphedema.

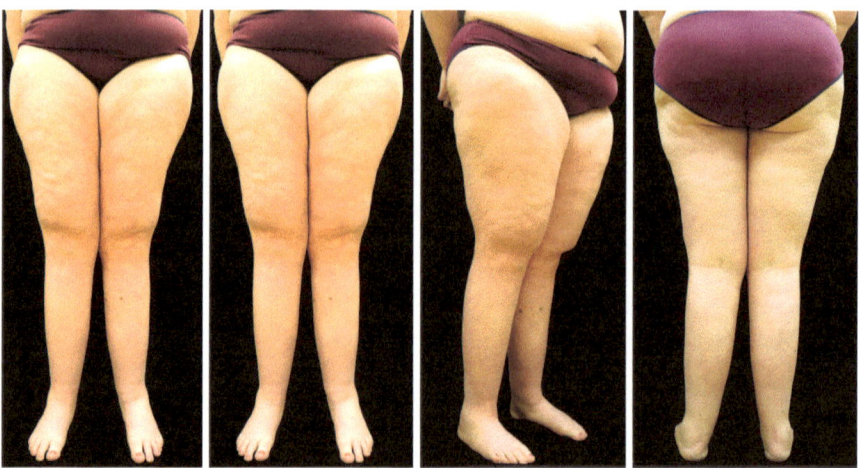

Fig. 1.18 Lipedema or combined lipo-lymphedema

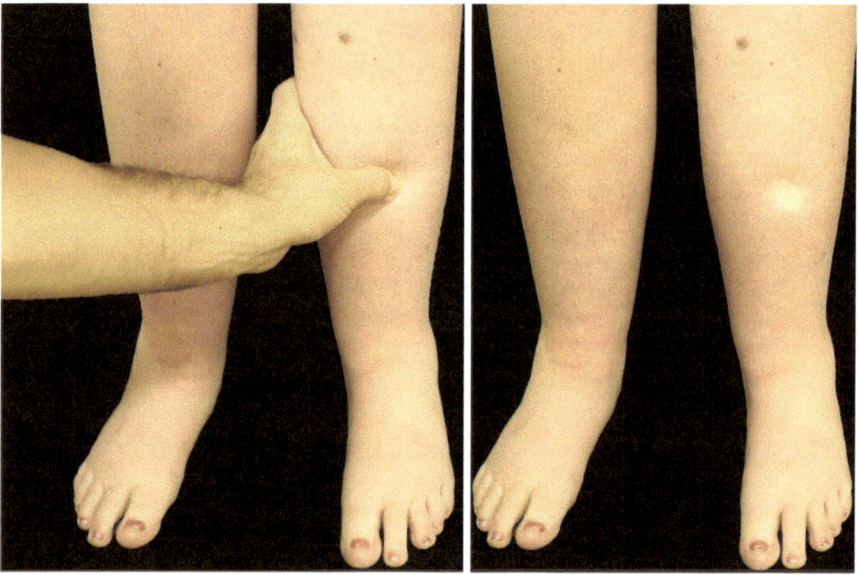

Fig. 1.19 Evidence of lipo lymphedema

▶ Edema in lipedema is rare.

Theory of Edema in the Adipocyte
There is another interesting theory on the subject of "edema in lipedema," and that is that the edema is IN the adipocyte (the fatty cell) that is, that the fat cells accumulate and store more water.

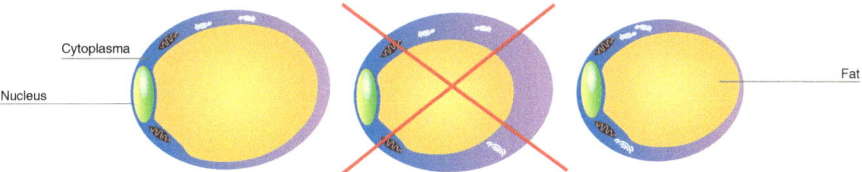

Fig. 1.20 Water retention in the cell

We have already discussed the cell structure of a fat cell in Sect. 1.2.1. Here we briefly summarize once again: A cell membrane separates the cell from the environment and within this, all components are surrounded by the cell water, the so-called cytoplasm. As the name "cell water" implies, the cytoplasm consists mainly of water. In the cytoplasm, we find the cell organelles, including the cell nucleus.

The fat cell stores fat in a fat vacuole. The ratio between nucleus and cytoplasm as well as cytoplasm and fat vacuole can be measured and determined. From this ratio, the cytoplasmic content can be measured and evaluated. There is currently no study that we are aware of that describes a difference in cell–cytoplasm ratio and proves increased water retention in a fat cell in lipedema. In the case of increased water storage, the cytoplasm ratio would be larger (Fig. 1.20). Rather, we suspect that a different development occurs: as the adipose tissue and thus the volume of the fat vacuole increases, the ratio of cytoplasm present could decrease.

Thus, the claim that a fat cell in lipedema stores water is rather false or at least not proven and thus baseless.

How does edema show up clinically? Indentable edema is more likely to be a sign of venous weakness, liver, cardiac, or renal disease. When pressure is applied to nondepressible edema, no dent remains in the tissue. Lymphedema may or may not be compressible, depending on the cause. The swelling or "edema" in classic lipedema is usually not compressible, so we talk about lipo-lymphedema.

We would like to show you an example from our practice that speaks against the edema theories presented. We perform many examinations of the lymphatic vessels in our lymphedema patients. For this purpose, we stain the lymphatic vessels to make them visible. By injecting a dye for lymphatic vessels, ICG (indocyanine green), in the area of the feet, we can visualize and examine the lymphatic vessels with the help of an infrared camera after a short waiting period. The dye is first injected into the space between the toes. After a short waiting period, the camera is used to examine the extent to which the lymphatic vessels absorb and remove the dye. In healthy people, the dye is taken up into lymphatic vessels and move along proximally without any sort of diffuse distribution in the tissue. In lymphedema, we regularly see a diffuse cloud or at least severe irregularities in the distribution pattern of the dye. We have also performed this examination in lipedema patients and have not seen any irregularities in the ICG uptake. This is purely an observation from our own experience.

▶   To determine whether you are suffering from edema, a simple examination is sufficient: press the tissue in the area of your front lower legs deeply. If a dent appears that does not disappear immediately but takes 2–3 s or longer, then it is possible that you are indeed suffering from edema, which is a rarity.

1.4   Pain

The indication of pain in the presence of a fat distribution disorder is THE decisive criterion for the diagnosis of "lipedema." Pain is the leading symptom of lipedema. It is important to note that related to pain, there is NO scientific evidence as to how the pain is actually triggered. What we do know for sure, however, is that it is located in the subcutaneous adipose tissue. Thousands of women suffer from this chronic pain in the buttocks, hips, legs, arms, and sometimes other regions. At the same time, we know quite different descriptions of pain in lipedema. The classical indicated pains are.

– pressure pain
– tearing pain
– strain pain
– touch pain and
– pain at rest.

It is typical for lipedema to be associated with hypersensitivity to touch and pain.

Pain Development
Although it has not been proven, the question is how the pain is caused. One theory is that the pain is caused by pressure in the tissues. Increased capillary permeability (permeability of the smallest blood vessels) to water and proteins causes the edema already described in the subcutaneous fat tissue. This is followed by pressure-induced tissue overstretching, which triggers pain via the activation of pain receptors.

For comparison, let us look at patients suffering from pure edema due to cardiac insufficiency, medication, or other diseases. These patients report NO form of pain in the areas of edema. Thus, we do not assume that it is the edema that triggers the pain in lipedema. Lymphedema patients also do not usually report pain, at least not in the same way as lipedema patients.

The theory is also questionable because there is usually no edema in lipedema.

▶   Pain is not caused by edema.

In contrast, the following mechanism is more plausible: In lipedema, there is an undersupply of oxygen in the adipose tissue. This triggers an inflammatory reaction, which in turn triggers vascular sprouting (fragile blood vessels), fibrosis (connective tissue proliferation). Furthermore, the lack of oxygen leads to increased fat cell death, which exceeds the natural death in the fat cell cycle. This observation was demonstrated in the laboratory via antibody assays. In the regions of oxygen deficiency, there was an increased number of phagocytes, which belong to the white blood cells, the leukocytes. Phagocytes are part of the body's innate immune response and may also be an indication of an inflammatory response. Other studies suggest an insidious, chronic inflammatory process.

Others suggest that excessive fat storage in fat cells causes a stress response, which in turn leads to the release of pro-inflammatory factors from the fat cells themselves and the immune cells in the adipose tissue. No matter how we spin it, everything points to an existing inflammatory response that irritates nerve receptors, which can trigger pain.

Described theories are a combination of scientifically proven facts, conjecture and hypotheses. That is all we can offer from our ranks on the subject of pain causation.

Complaints in the sense of pain often occur in the later stages. Nevertheless, we see sufferers in very early stages with markedly severe pain. Consequently, pain intensity does not seem to correlate with disease progression.

▶　　The visual stage of the disease "lipedema" does not correlate with pain intensity. Although the pain is usually pronounced in later stages, we also see women in early stages with very severe pain.

1.5　A Chronic-Progressive Course?

Let us turn our attention to another often postulated claim concerning the course of lipedema. Many speak of a chronic-progressive evolution. Chronic-progressive means that the existing lipedema continuously and inexorably worsens. Very often, it is precisely this fear of uncontrolled and permanent progression of lipedema that brings those affected to us. These fears are fueled by Internet portals or media who also propagate a cure through holistic liposuction. This claim is additionally underlined by extreme patient examples, which we all know from the internet, alongside texts like "Who wants to end up like that" all these rattling the conscience of those affected. This is, of course, pure nonsense.

If we break this assertion down into its component parts, we are talking about the words chronic and progressive.

Chronic refers to the period. If lipedema with its symptoms is present for more than 6 months, we can safely speak of chronic disease.

Progressive or progressive means "progressing." If we put the words "chronic" and "progressive" together again, then this is meant to describe a long-lasting disease in which the manifestation of the symptoms increases continuously over a long period. However, this course does not apply to the disease "lipedema." However, from our point of view lipedema must be understood as a "disease that progresses chronically in episodes." What does this small but subtle difference mean?

Let's look again at the development of lipedema: lipohypertrophy develops into lipedema (pain is added). Lipedema can remain at this stage for years or forever. Often, there are one or more relapses (hormonal changes), which then aggravate the lipedema. Nevertheless, the fact remains that lipedema does not worsen in every patient. We know some affected people who are 80 years old and have been in stage I for what feels like an eternity. It should be noted that the stage does not indicate the severity of the symptoms.

▶   Lipedema is NOT a chronic progressive disease, but a chronic relapsing disease.

Nevertheless, in clinical practice, we see massive numbers of patients with lipedema that increase over the years. The reason for this is either the aggravation of the existing hormonal harmony (estrogen-progestin) or progressive obesity, which is wrongly distributed due to the congenital fat distribution disorder aggravating the situation.

There is one thing that everyone is sure to agree on: if weight gain occurs in the presence of an existing disproportion in the sense of lipohypertrophy (without pain) or lipedema (with pain), this will always have a negative effect on the affected regions. This fact has been known since its first description in 1940.

1.6   Obesity and Lipedema

The number of massively overweighted patients we see in our ambulatory center is steadily increasing. As we will see, there is a link between lipedema and obesity. Worldwide, obesity has increased dramatically in recent years, which also explains the significant increase in lipedema cases.

Obesity does not have a good reputation worldwide and is often associated with own failure, lack of discipline, loss of control, and many other prejudices. Many of us know how difficult it is to control our weight or even lose a few more pounds. No one can count on help from the food industry, which contributes quite a bit to the calamity. Many resign themselves over time, and the frustration grows greater and greater with each failed attempt to control weight. We are all human and when we fail—perhaps without realizing it—we look for explanations. When we fail at something, we like to subconsciously explain to ourselves that no one can do it and/or there must be some other reason. If we then encounter the thesis that you can't lose weight with fat legs, we gladly accept it and feel a sense of relief. For this reason, the statement: "Whoever suffers from lipedema cannot lose weight" has become quite persistent and has even arrived in the professional literature. And that's exactly how convinced those affected tell us in our consultations—without knowing where this insight comes from. We have not seen any proof for this thesis until today.

Of course, we cannot make it so simple for ourselves and will illuminate the connection with "weight loss and shape change" in lipedema in detail in Chap. 3, "Treatment of lipedema" and put our statement into perspective.

Some medical colleagues also use lipedema for themselves. If you don't know how to treat it, dubbing it "lipedema" comes in handy, true to the motto: "There's nothing we can do about it—that's what everyone wants to hear and that's that."

"I'm not fat, I suffer from lipedema." I stand behind this statement, as long as we are talking about sufferers who are not extremely obese. For those who are extremely obese, it should correctly read, "I suffer from obesity and lipedema." Consequently, my first statement applies only to sufferers who are of normal weight or only slightly overweight. A fat distribution disorder in favor of the legs with an otherwise slim figure has nothing to do with "being fat."

Obesity or adiposity (from Latin adeps = fat) is a nutritional and metabolic disease. Obesity is characterized by an increase in body fat above normal levels. Obesity was classified as a disease by the World Health Organization many years ago. There is even talk of a so-called obesity epidemic.

▶ Obesity is a widespread disease.

Obesity is not "a few kilos too much," but a significant excess of body fat tissue. This condition can cause a whole range of diseases that not only significantly reduce the quality of life but also shorten life expectancy.

When it comes to obesity, it is important to be able to estimate your own body weight. To do this, one must be able to put the excess weight in perspective. To assess obesity, the BMI (body mass index) has become widely accepted.

$$BMI = \frac{\text{body weight [kg]}}{\text{body height} \times \text{body size} \left[m^2 \right]}$$

If the BMI value is around 25 kg/m², there is little risk of developing secondary diseases in the future due to being underweight or overweight. On the other hand, if the BMI is around 27 kg/m2, you have the highest life expectancy ever.

Did you know that being underweight is much more harmful to our health than being overweight? Being underweight is associated with diseases of the body much faster than being overweight. For a person who is 160 cm tall and weighs 60 kg, being 50% overweight, that is, a bodyweight of 90 kg (BMI 35.19 kg/m²), is harmful in the long term, but being 50% underweight, that is, a bodyweight of 30 kg (BMI 11.72 kg/m²), is life-threatening and virtually fatal. From a BMI of 13 kg/m2, inpatient treatment is required due to severe malnutrition and danger to life. Anorexia is defined as a BMI < 17.5 kg/m² or a bodyweight less than 15% below normal.

In normal-weight men, the amount of regular depot fat is about 15 kg; in women, it is 15–20 kg. If the percentage of fat in body weight exceeds 20% in men and 30% in women, obesity is present.

From a BMI of 25–29.9 kg/m², we speak of being overweight. This is widely encountered in the population. It is assumed that far more than 50% of all German citizens suffer from overweight or a more severe form. By definition, we speak of obesity (adiposity) from a BMI of 30 kg/m². All higher BMI values are then only used to distinguish the severity of obesity (Table 1.2, Fig. 1.21).

Table 1.2 Weight classes depending on BMI (according to WHO classification)

BMI in kg/m2	Type
<24	<24 underweight
24–27	Normal weight
28–29	Slightly overweight
30–34	Obesity/obesity grade I
35–39	Obesity/obesity grade II
>40	Obesity/obesity grade III

Fig. 1.21 Obesity

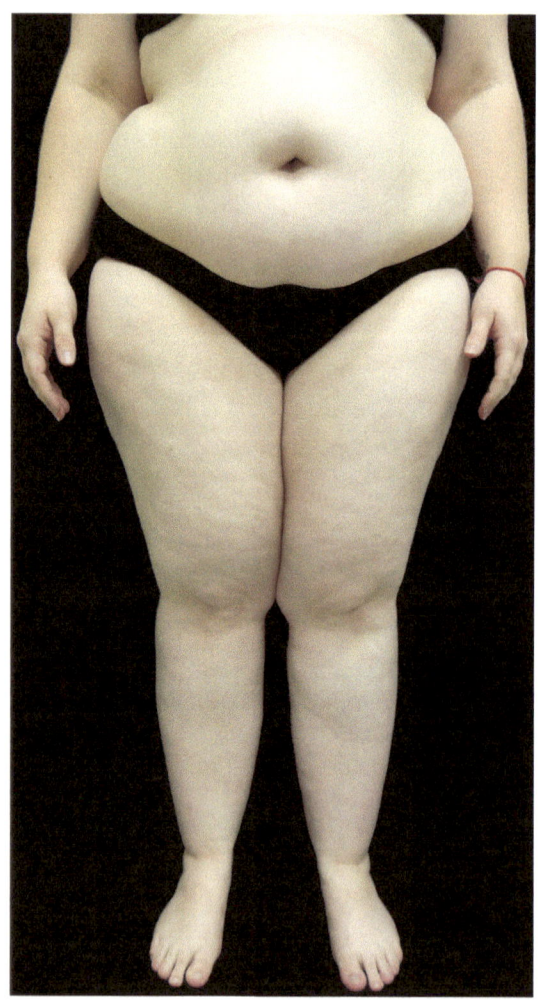

A BMI of 30–34 kg/m² is referred to as obesity grade I, a BMI of 35–39 kg/m² is referred to as obesity grade II, and a BMI of >40 kg/m² corresponds to obesity grade III. The higher the obesity, the greater.

A BMI of 30–34 kg/m² is referred to as obesity grade I, a BMI of 35–39 kg/m² is referred to as obesity grade II, and a BMI of >40 kg/m² corresponds to obesity grade III. The higher the obesity, the greater the risk for secondary diseases and a shortened life expectancy.

Possible Causes

Obesity develops whenever energy intake exceeds energy consumption. There can be very different causes for this.

▶ Due to the high number of overweight or obese lipedema sufferers, the number of normal weight sufferers is underrepresented. There is no scientific evidence that lipedema leads to obesity.

Very decisive in the development of obesity seems to be the genetic factor, that is, the inherited predisposition, to obesity. Very rarely, only one gene is responsible for present obesity. In these cases, we speak of rare monogenic forms (i.e., one gene). Much more frequently, there is an interaction of several genes (polygenic forms). Each interacting gene then contributes to obesity. Targets of these genes can be appetite control, weight regulation, energy balance, hunger-satiety regulation, and food intake. It is believed (twin studies) that our body weight is about 70% determined by our genes.

▶ Obesity has many underlying causes. Approximately 70% of our body weight is predetermined by our genes.

Obesity can also be triggered by metabolic disease. Examples here are an underactive thyroid gland or an overactive adrenal gland. It is equally possible for obesity to occur as a result of surgery on a body gland or the brain. Another reason for weight gain may be medication use. Examples include the use of cortisone, hormone preparations, and psychotropic drugs such as antidepressants.

▶ Only in a few sufferers are metabolic diseases, surgery, and medication use responsible for weight gain (estimated at 1 in 100 sufferers).

Weight and Age

Middle-aged women are a special case. Almost 2/third of women aged 40–59 and about 3/fourth of women over 60 in the United States are overweight with a BMI over 27 kg/m². After the age of 40, there is an average annual weight gain of about 0.7 kg. These changes lead to a decrease in both rest- and activity-related energy expenditure. Therefore, aging leads to weight gain unless there is a compensatory change in dietary habits and physical activity.

In addition, there are symptoms such as mood swings, loss of drive and motivation, sleep disturbances, and the classic complaints of the musculoskeletal system. The preceding symptoms also support further weight gain.

There is a change in body fat distribution from the premenopausal gynoid pattern (pear type) to the postmenopausal android pattern (apple type).

Fat Distribution

Apple type and Pear type? That is only figuratively speaking! If we look at the gender-specific characteristics of fat distribution, we often see in men belly-emphasized fat tissue storage with fat deposits around the internal organs, but also in the subcutaneous fat tissue on the abdomen. Here we speak of the central type, the "apple type." The situation is different in women, in whom the adipose tissue is already located to a greater extent in the buttock–hip area for genetic reasons. This distribution is referred to as the "pear type" (Fig. 1.22).

The transition from pre- to postmenopausal is often also the time when lipohypertrophy first develops, painfully changes to lipedema, or when preexisting lipedema worsens. Lipedema adipose tissue, often referred to as "lip fat," is often initially found in the bulbous regions of obese individuals. We try to avoid the term

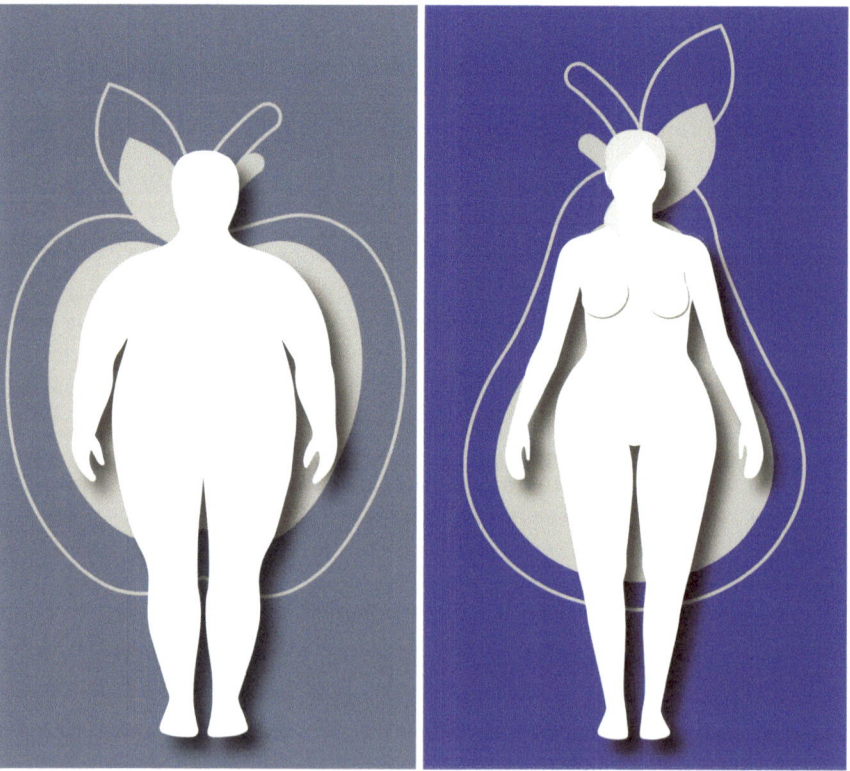

Fig. 1.22 Apple and pear type

"lipid fat"because it suggests that one can distinguish adipose tissue of lipedema from healthy adipose tissue with the naked eye or via ultrasound, when in fact only some immunohistochemical markers are able to do so. In only slightly overweight and slender women, however, we often find the fat distribution disorder in the area of the entire lower extremity, often as a so-called columnar leg, where the entire leg contour resembles a column (Fig. 1.23).

The male apple type is much more harmful than the female pear type. Especially dangerous is the abdominal fat, that is, the fat around the organs. Fatification of the abdomen—and this has been scientifically proven—has a detrimental effect specifically on the function of the internal organs. For women, an abdominal girth of 80 cm or more and for men, 94 cm or more is considered harmful (Fig. 1.24).

▶   Waist circumference is associated with the amount of "belly fat" and is closely related to cardiovascular disease.

Calorie Turnover
As already mentioned in Sects. 1.2.3 and 1.2.6, we often do not use as much energy as we consume. The surplus is simply not utilized but is stored in the adipose tissue. Moreover, if one suffers from an estrogen receptor distribution disorder, as is suspected in lipedema, even less energy is probably sufficient to store fat.

In the past, storing fat was necessary for survival, because we didn't know when we'd next have something to eat. We built up a bacon coat for the winter as heat insulation and energy storage. Nowadays, this is different. Our food supply is

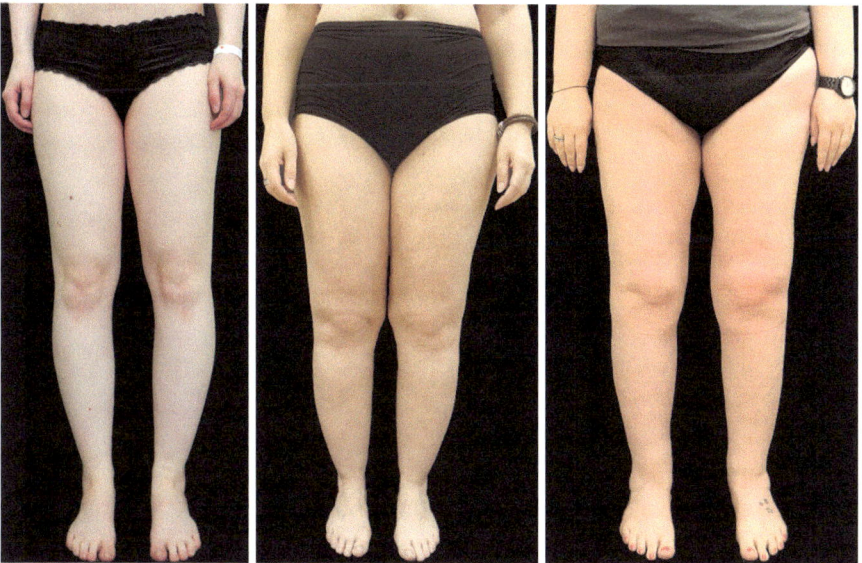

Fig. 1.23 Examples of different column legs

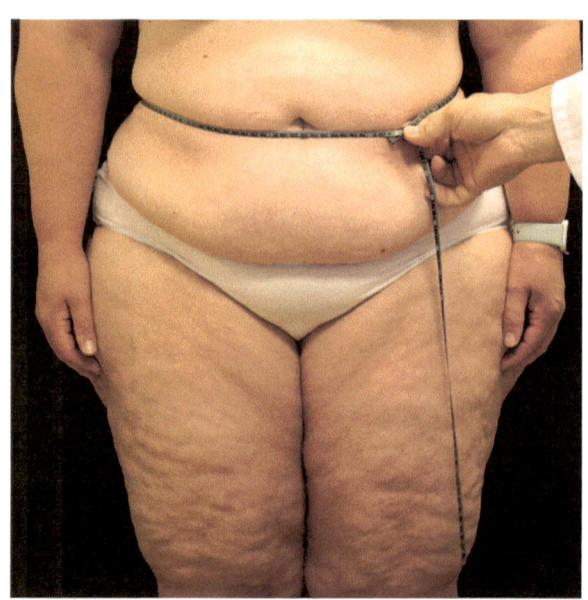

Fig. 1.24 Circumference measurement at the waist

secure. Nevertheless, our body still thinks and works according to the old principles. Eat whenever possible! For us humans, the development into prosperity simply happened too fast for our behavior to have been able to adapt through evolution. Our eating behavior, thus, lags far behind the current supply. We must therefore actively take countermeasures to change our behavior.

Our daily total caloric expenditure is on average 2300 kcal and consists of a basal metabolic rate and activity metabolic rate. The basal metabolic rate can be roughly estimated. Multiply the body weight by 24 and you have a very good approximation.

▶   The caloric basal metabolic rate can be roughly estimated using the formula: Bodyweight × 24.

But if you want to know more about it here in detail:

The basal metabolic rate is the amount of energy required by the body at rest and at indifference temperature (28 °C) during 1 day (24 h) to maintain its function. It is, so to speak, the "standby turnover." Of course, many factors play a determining role in the basal metabolic rate, for example,

– Age.
– Gender.
– Bodyweight.
– Body size.
– Proportion of muscle mass.

- Ambient temperature and thermal insulation by clothing as well as.
- General state of health.

To calculate the basal metabolic rate, the "Harris–Benedict formula"has proven itself. The value is not exact, but a very good approximation to the real basal metabolic rate. In the basal metabolic rate, the brain, heart, and kidneys have the highest demand for energy.

For women:

$$\text{Basal metabolic rate} / (\frac{kcal}{24\,h} = 655,1 + (9,6 \times \text{body weight}[kg])$$
$$+ (1,8 \times \text{body height}[cm]) - (4,7 \times age[years])$$

Although not many men will read it, here the formula for comparison:

$$\text{Basal metabolic rate} / (\frac{kcal}{24\,h} = 66,47 + (13,7 \times \text{body weight}[kg])$$
$$+ (5 \times \text{body height}[cm]) - (6,8 \times age[years])$$

If we now go into further detail, we can name the energy metabolism of various tissue components (Table 1.3). Although the brain accounts for only about 2% of body weight, it consumes quite a lot of our daily basal metabolic rate. We can roughly say that 20% of the basal metabolic rate is consumed by the brain. 500 g of brain mass consumes about 110 kcal per day. Our brain has an approximate weight of 1500 g, which makes a brain calorie basal metabolic rate of 330 kcal per day. The special thing about the brain is that it can only burn sugar and takes it directly from food.

Kidney tissue consumes about 200 kcal per day. One kidney weighs about 130 g. 500 g of muscle mass consume 6 kcal, 500 g of fat 2 kcal per day.

▶   Our brain burns an average of 330 kcal per day and can only utilize sugar.

Power Conversion

Our activity or power metabolism is the amount of energy that we burn in 1 day with our body. This turnover is mainly generated by brain and muscle activity (work, leisure, sport). To calculate the conduction metabolic rate, we use the PAL value ("Physical Activity Level"; Table 1.4; Fig. 1.25).

Table 1.3 Energy metabolism by tissue

Tissue	Mass (g)	Consumption per day [kcal]
Brain	1500	330
Kidney tissue	130	200
Muscle tissue	500	6
Fat	500	2

Table 1.4 PAL value

Factor	Activity	Example
0,95	Sleeping	Night rest
1,2–1,3	Sitting, lying	Seniors, bedridden people
1,4–1,5	Sitting, little physical activity	Desk workers
1,6–1,7	Predominantly sitting, walking, standing	Pupils, students, bus drivers
1,8–1,9	Predominantly walking and standing	Salespersons, waiters, mail carriers
2,0–2,4	Physical work	Construction workers, farmers, loggers, athletes

Recommendation of daily energy intake in kilocalories (kcal)						
Adults	**PAL-value 1.4**		**PAL-value 1.6**		**PAL-value 1.8**	
Gender	male	female	male	female	male	female
AGE						
19 - 25 years	2400	1900	2800	2200	3100	2500
25 - 51 years	2300	1800	2700	2100	3000	2400
51 - 65 years	2200	1700	2500	2000	2800	2200
65 and older	2100	1700	2500	1900	2800	2100

Fig. 1.25 PAL values

For this purpose, the factors are multiplied by the respective number of hours and then added. To obtain a daily average, this number must be divided by 24. To determine the total energy requirement, the daily average is multiplied by the basal metabolic rate. The result is the average total energy requirement (Fig. 1.26). The daily total calorie requirement thus varies from individual to individual.

Let us now take a look at the calories' consumption of other activities: We assume a person weighing 70 kg and the calories consumption within 1 h (Table 1.5).

Energy Intake and Eating Behavior

Let's look now at energy intake and how we supply ourselves with energy. The "how" may sound strange at first, but our eating habits are more unfavorable than ever before. We are talking here about our eating behavior. We eat on the side, standing up, and often stressed—all negative characteristics.

Many eat only in between and unconsciously, for which they should not be blamed. In a big city, the most appetizing treats are held under our noses virtually every 50 m. Not only in the pedestrian zones but also on the roadways we find inviting fast-food snacks against ravenous appetite. It's often difficult to resist as we walk by, and if we don't find anything as we pass by, we subconsciously know that an online ordering food center won't let us down. This gives us added confidence

PAL values for different activities

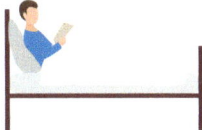

PAL value 1.2 -1.3
For a person who is exclusively sitting or lying

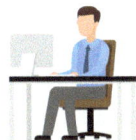

PAL value 1.4 -1.6
For people with mainly sedentary work

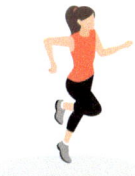

PAL value 2.0 - 2.4
For people with very active leisure design

Fig. 1.26   Calorie requirements by activity level

Table 1.5   Calorie consumption within 1 h

Activity	Kcal/h
Weightlifting	224
Water gymnastics	149
Cycling (moderate)	260
Rowing (moderate)	260
Cross trainer	335
Billiards	93
Golf	130
Walking (6,4 km/h)	167
Jogging (12 km/h)	465
Gardening	167
Sleeping	23
Cooking	93
TV	28
In standing in a queue	47
Playing with the kids	147
Wallpapering/painting	167
Computer work	51
Counter work	65
Forestry worker	298

that we won't go hungry. Conveniently, we kill two birds with one stone with delivery services: first, we get the food delivered and don't have to "pick or hunt" like we used to, because that also used to burn a very large percentage of calories. Second, we don't even have to go to the trouble of preparing it! What a luxury we live in. What we don't know is what's really in the products. Besides flavor enhancers, there are huge amounts of fats and sugars in the products. Therefore, our food is often unbalanced and one-sided. Vegetables, fruits, and other things are completely missing in many such items. Ready-made meals are often no better (Fig. 1.27).

We haven't even discussed two major calorie bombs yet: sweets and soft drinks. In Germany, around 31 kg of sweets are bought and eaten per capita every year, and

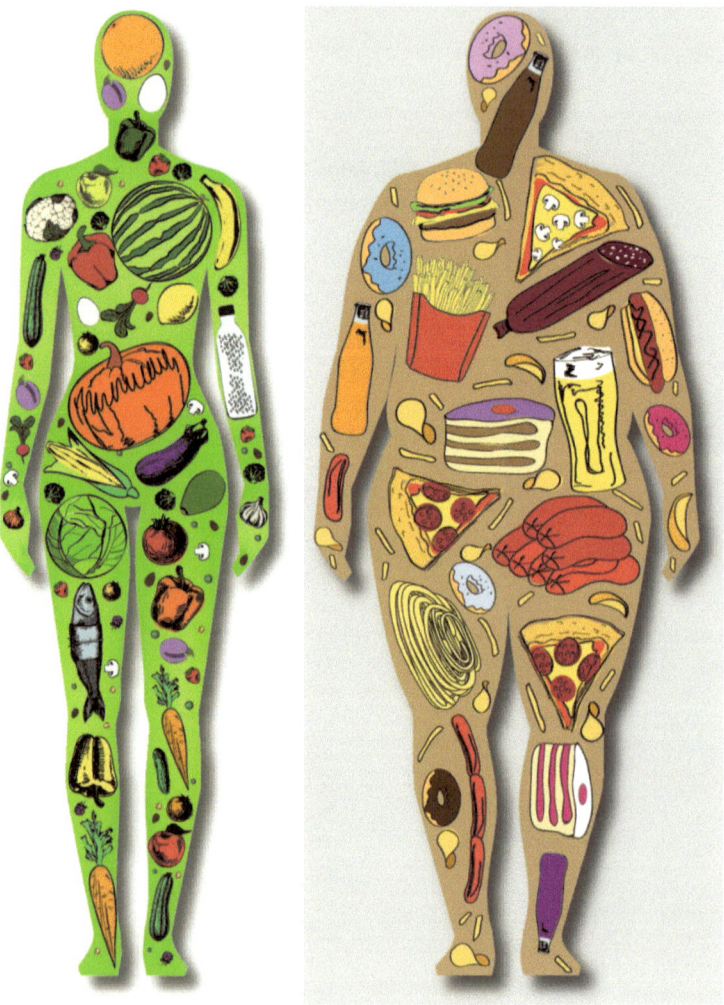

Fig. 1.27 Healthy and unhealthy food

on average, every German drinks around 133 liters of soft drinks, the liquid sugar bombs, per year. In the USA, on the other hand, 195 l are drunk per person. A truly frighteningly high figure.

Expectations of one's own role and social stress are further factors. Eating disorders of various kinds are often present. Obesity due to a psychological cause (so-called psychogenic obesity) is not in itself a distinct clinical picture, although a very high number of people suffer from this cause of obesity.

However, many of those affected are not even aware of the psychological background of their suffering. Most often, binge eating is used to regulate emotions. Often, people with psychogenic obesity use food to cope with unpleasant or disturbing feelings such as loneliness, stress, anger, boredom, overwhelm, sadness, disregard, or trauma (whether violent or sexual). Sometimes weight gain is said to unconsciously cause one to acquire a "protective armor" and thus lose attractiveness.

In many cases, those affected are internally oversensitive and vulnerable. Eating is used as a way of regulating feelings. Many speak of so-called substitute satisfaction in these situations.

In addition, there are negative habits: Some eat when they are stressed, others when they are successful, and others eat throughout—whether at work or on the road—a little candy here and a piece of cake there.

Did you know that with age the body learns to digest food better? Therefore, the nutrient yield in old age is better than in youth. Another reason why we get by with less food as we age.

Finally, we have the suffering topic of smoking. Many people try to quit smoking, especially nowadays when smoking is becoming more and more frowned upon and unpopular. The undesirable side effect is an increase in body weight. The exact reasons why we gain weight when we stop smoking are many. In addition to an abolished appetite control, the "substitute drug candy" is often to blame.

Energy Consumption and Lifestyle
As with energy supply, we are also dealing with a multilayered issue when it comes to energy consumption. Our own lifestyle plays a major role. This is often inactive and passive. Even short distances are covered by a car. Hunting and gathering are long gone. We live in a society of comfort, in which we allow ourselves to be entertained.

Psychosocial factors also play a role here. The influence of an intact family (nuclear family) and intact family life, as well as friends and circle of friends, are important for our activity.

Do you walk the stairs or take the elevator? Even up to the fifth floor? What about sports? Do you go to the gym or have you only been paying your contributions for years?

Our very own biology doesn't help us to keep our weight either because in principle we only have two programs inside us. One program tells us to eat whenever we find something to eat (we just discussed that). The second program tells us to conserve as much energy as possible, that is, to move minimally to stay at maximum strength. That's why we feel so comfortable "chilling." In the past, at least, we burned energy hunting and gathering. Today we reach for the tablet or cell phone. We prefer cars and other means of transportation and are happy to leave the bike behind. For the most part, walking no longer finds a place in our fast-paced times. Our workplaces often involve a lot of sitting, and you can already tell we're "chilling through life." One could cite many more examples here that would underline our "chill mentality."

In addition, there is the psyche, which we will discuss in detail in the following section. The background is that lipedema sufferers, who suffer from chronic pain, exclusion, and strong dissatisfaction with their appearance, are often plagued by depressive mood or actual depression.

1.7 Complaints and Effects of Lipedema

We have already talked about pathomechanism, which is still unknown to us, and obesity, which often occurs in combination. Now it is time to talk about the symptoms and the course of the disease "lipedema." Since lipedema can be a chameleon, there are statements we can make in general, but likewise, there are always exceptions.

Typically, lipohypertrophy starts in the area of the lower extremities (incl. Buttocks and hips). Accordingly, it is often seen at the first moment merely visually: "Something is wrong here." Subsequently, those affected notice a feeling of heaviness in the legs and only then, in the further course of the disease and the later stages, there is a feeling of tension and pain in the area of the affected regions.

Most often we see that lipedema starts in the lower half of the body and then moves to the upper part of the body.

▶ Typically, lipedema begins after the onset of lipohypertrophy in the lower extremity. Only in the later stages can the upper extremity be affected.

We see a wide range of sensitivity to touch and touch pain in our patients. For many, it is even the smallest touches and strokes that can trigger an unpleasant feeling or even pain. This often leads to a withdrawal from the own relationship with the resulting further conflict-building sites.

From our clinical experience, further typical complaints are feeling tension or pain in the sense of pressure pain, touch pain, or tearing pain. Mostly the complaints occur during the day and bring restlessness in the legs. In many cases, the pain is most pronounced in the evening. If there is temporary or permanent edema, then a worsening of the symptoms with an increase in edema during the day is often reported.

The curious thing about our current system is that if you suffer from a fat distribution disorder, you are only recognized as "sick" if you have pain. If one has no pain, one is considered healthy. In fact, one is treated only when one reaches a certain visual stage, but this has nothing to do with pain. If one does not see any-thing visually or if one can only rudimentarily recognize a fat distribution disorder and the patient states severe pain, she is still considered healthy (or a spinner, which is even worse). But even if both criteria apply, that is, a fat distribution disorder is associated with pain and the patient is overweight, she will not have an easy time with treatment.

We see very many affected persons—whether normal or overweight—who do not suffer from pain but a restriction of their mobility. Regardless of the visual stage, in our view, a restriction of movement is pathological above a certain level (Fig. 1.28).

It is often deforming fat pads on the inner thighs and knees (Fig. 1.29) that cause restricted movement. In addition to a leg malposition, these lead to increased

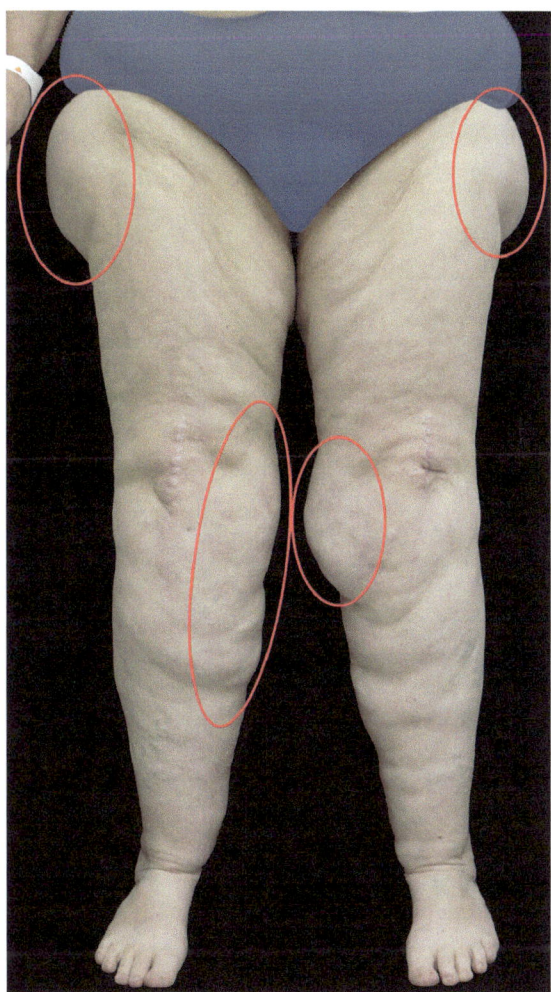

Fig. 1.28 Movement restriction due to excess skin and adipose tissue

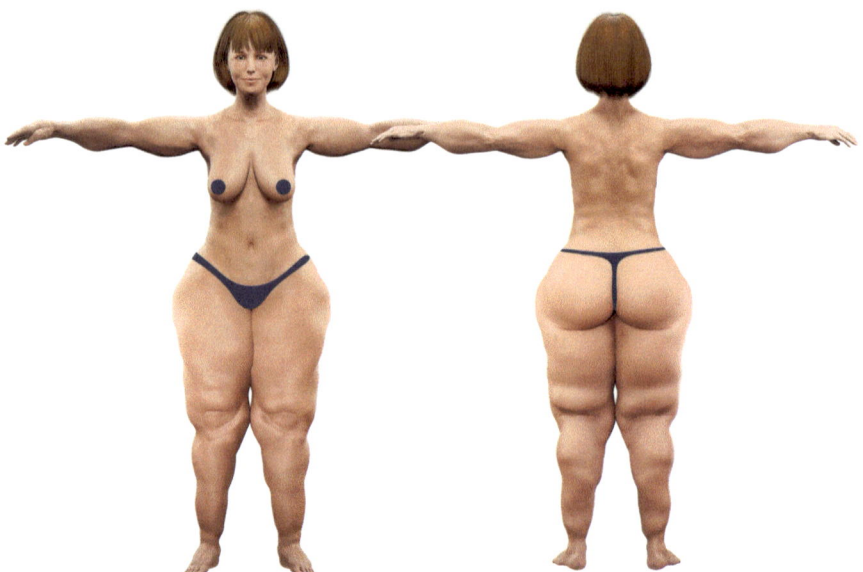

Fig. 1.29 Deforming fat pads/lipedema type 4 stage III

sweating, redness, and itching. Often, the affected persons cannot do sports and are less resilient both at work and in their private lives. If skin flaps are present, moist chambers propagating fungal infections can form in these intercutaneous furrows.

It is unfair if we recognize a fat distribution disorder as a disease only with pain. There are definitely complaints that can be associated with a fat distribution disorder and thus also have a disease value (and we have not yet talked about the psychological burden).

Affected persons with a fat distribution disorder without pain, but with a restriction of movement due to the fat masses and skin flaps, are entitled to treatment like everyone else. Certainly, one must ask oneself which treatment would be the right one in these cases. For this, an individual therapy plan must be created.

Be it lipohypertrophy or lipedema: many affected people also suffer psychologically from the consequences of their external appearance. Often, this aspect is given far too little attention! From the very beginning, however, we have to distinguish between a burden limiting the feeling of being alive or the quality of life and a manifest, severe psychological disorder.

Many, especially physicians and administrators such as health insurers, know only one or the other. We have a different view of things; from our perspective, there are many intermediate levels.

The lightest form of a psychological burden (and in our eyes, it is not even a burden) is the subliminal dissatisfaction concerning external body appearance caused by lipedema or lipohypertrophy. We are not talking here about a body dysmorphic disorder, which is present when there is a pathological perception of one's body image, but about psychologically stable women who are simply a little more than dissatisfied with one or another part of their body.

If we go one step further, those affected often describe a "discomfort" with the external appearance. Although the "problem" is not always completely comprehensible objectively, it is recognizable and identifiable. Those affected are somewhat more isolated but still very active socially, however refusing to go to the swimming pools or the beach, so places where they are forced to expose their body.

Higher suffering pressure usually exists in patients with a comprehensible objective disproportion. Those affected often withdraw in social life and also in relationships. A depressive mood and mood swings are often described.

In the case of pronounced deformities, we often see a very strong restriction of the quality of life up to withdrawal from the relationship and the social environment. A very high level of suffering prevails, the entire life is restricted, with depression and other mental illnesses requiring specialized treatment.

These psychological components now have two effects: One is a lack of drive and thus a withdrawal from sports and general activities. Less exercise automatically reduces the daily calorie consumption, but at the same time, there is another effect, the reduction of muscle mass having a negative effect on the daily caloric basal metabolic rate. The second effect is the so-called "frustration" or "emotional" eating. In this case, food is used to process emotions—a vicious circle that is difficult to break, and one that nutritional psychology deals with intensively. Sufferers often reduce themselves to their lipohypertrophy or lipedema and feel stigmatized accordingly. "Everyone stares at me and thinks I'm just fat."

In all of the described mental states, the affected persons can additionally suffer from pain. However, let's assume that there is no pain, neither in the legs nor in the arms. Now everyone must decide for themselves to what extent we have a social responsibility to also take care of these affected persons and to reintegrate them into our society.

Let us now deal with manifest lipedema patients. More than 60% of women with lipedema have a mental illness. These psychological conditions are not necessarily related to lipedema but have usually arisen independently of it beforehand. The reasons for such mental illnesses are often other, for example, physical illnesses, motivational disorders, burnout, depression, trauma in the sense of violence and sexual abuse, family situations such as separations, personality disorders, and so on. Often the underlying illness is an eating disorder. This is often disregarded or at least the aspect of "eating disorder" is often not taken seriously enough.

Here, a mixture often takes place and lipedema is blamed for this situation. Only in a small proportion of <5% does a manifest mental illness develop due to lipedema.

Lipedema with its pain, restricted movement, and visual dissatisfaction certainly leads to psychological stress with a reduction in self-esteem, withdrawal, and ultimately a reduction in the general quality of life. It is certainly impossible to predict which factors must come together in what way and with what intensity for a manifest mental disorder to develop. It is the combination of the factors whose weighting and duration of action enter into the trigger mechanism.

Over 30% of those affected by lipedema suffer from depression and severe mood swings.

Clearly, our mental and physical condition influences our performance. If we suffer from pathological, already existing or newly developed psychological impairments, and chronic pain is added to this, this can be compared to a continuous and slow, drop-by-drop erosion of a stone. In addition, there are physical complaints. Restricted mobility and reduced physical resilience further add to the already difficult situation.

Statements such as "I got depressed because of my lipedema" should be formulated with caution in this context. Perhaps depression or depressive mood was already present before the onset of lipedema. We agree with many colleagues and consider lipedema to be a factor that can support or aggravate a psychological condition.

There is scientific work that proves that there is a link between obesity and depression. As we already know, obesity is present in a large number of lipedema sufferers. Now the question here is which came first: depression or obesity. There is evidence for both directions here. Studies have shown that the risk of developing obesity increases with depression. Likewise, the other way around, it has been shown that obesity can lead to depression. Whichever way you look at it, one thing is clear: both promote the further development of existing or developing obesity and lipedema.

1.8   Appearance, Stages, Classifications, and Course

If lipohypertrophy or lipedema is present, the entire body must be considered for an appropriate assessment of its severity. The overall picture of disproportion, body weight, and body length must be taken into account. However, these morphological parameters are only descriptive of the disease and illustrate the current situation. They in no way reflect the course or severity of the disease.

The same problem applies to the currently used classification of lipedema into types and stages. The type describes the affected areas of the body, that is, which regions of the body are affected by lipedema. The stage describes the manifestation in the respective area. It is therefore purely a description of the external form.

We noticed in our clinical practice that there is always confusion on this subject, not least because there are several possible classifications. Therefore, we briefly present the individual type classifications below.

We will start with what is probably the most common type of classification (Table 1.6). Type I, which is often erroneously referred as "breech deformity."

Table 1.6 Classification of lipedema types

Type	Region
Type I	Hips and thighs are affected.
Type II	Lipedema extends to the knees.
Type III	The entire legs from hips to ankle are affected.
Type IV	The legs and arms are affected.

"Rider pants" deformity per se is a painless fat distribution disorder/lipohypertrophy and describes a fat distribution disorder in the hip–thigh region. In type II, this finding extends further toward the knee, while in type III, the entire legs are affected from the hips to the ankle region. In type IV, the legs and arms are affected (Fig. 1.30).

Another classification, mostly used by physicians, is that according to Herpertz. Here, lipedema is classified according to the affected localization and also named accordingly (Table 1.7).

The disadvantage of these two classifications is that no attention is paid to the buttocks, although in our clinical experience this area is also a frequently affected problem zone (Fig. 1.31).

The stage reflects the extent or the progress of the disease. Depending on the user, 3 or 4 stages are distinguished. The inflammatory reaction in the area of the adipose tissue is held responsible for the different manifestations of lipedema in the various stages. In the early stages, the adipose tissue is therefore often soft and loose, while in the later stages, it tends to be firmer and more nodular. Lipo-lymphedema is the last and also, fortunately, the rarest stage. It develops due to damage to the capillaries in combination with high tissue pressure, which severely restricts lymphatic drainage (Table 1.8; Fig. 1.32).

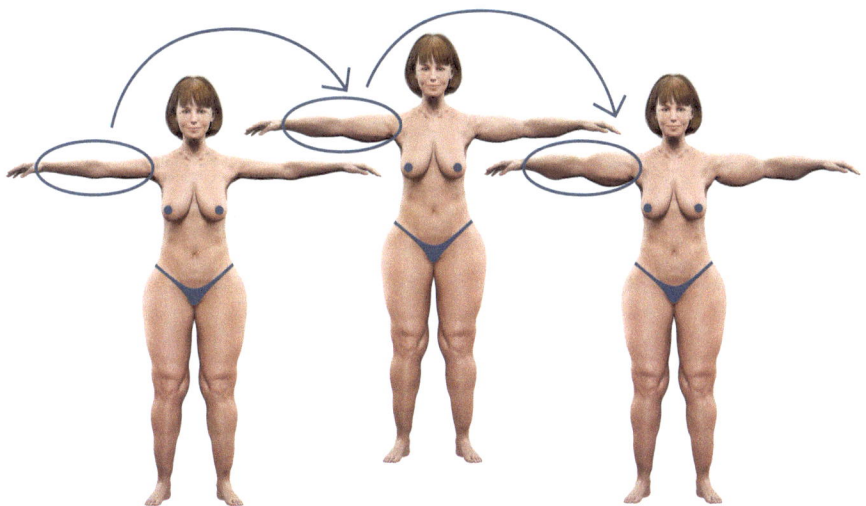

Fig. 1.30 Change of arms at different stages

Table 1.7 Lipedema according to affected localization

Legs	Arms
Upper leg type	Upper arm type
Whole leg type	Whole arm type
Lower leg type	Lower arm type

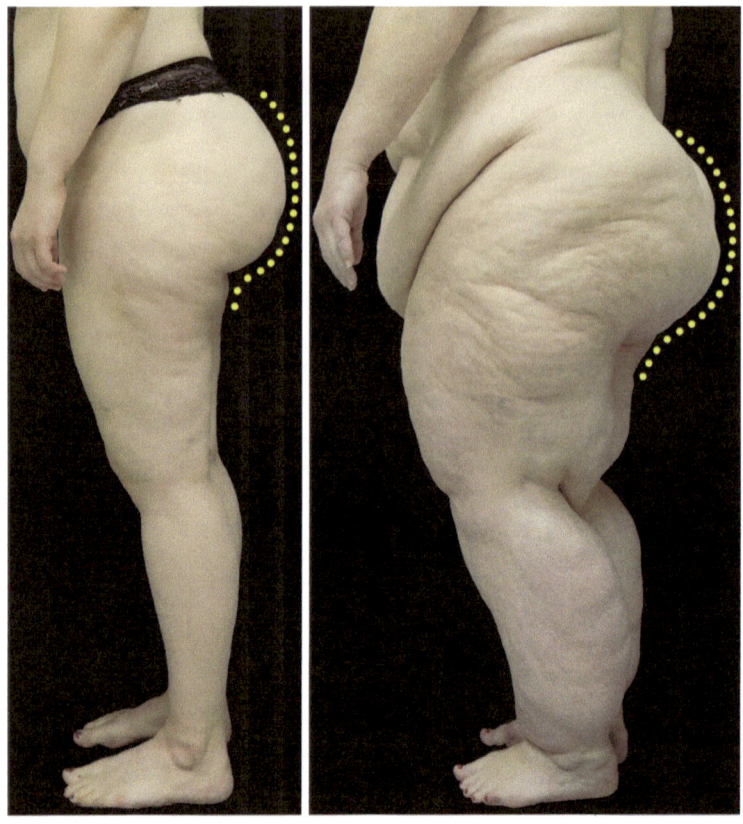

Fig. 1.31 Different manifestations of lipedema of the buttocks

Table 1.8 Staging of lipedema

Stage	Expression
Stage I	Smooth skin, fine nodular fat
Stage II	Uneven skin, coarse nodular fat
Stage III	Skin-fat flaps with deforming character, coarse tissue
Stage IV	Lipo-lymphoedema

Some others distinguish only three stages, and still others additionally distinguish the different tissue layers and include other features in their classification. There are actually very wide variations here. In the German guidelines on lipedema, only three stages are described.

Here is a citation from the currently available S1 Guideline on Lipedema (as of 10/2015), found on the website: https://www.awmf.org:

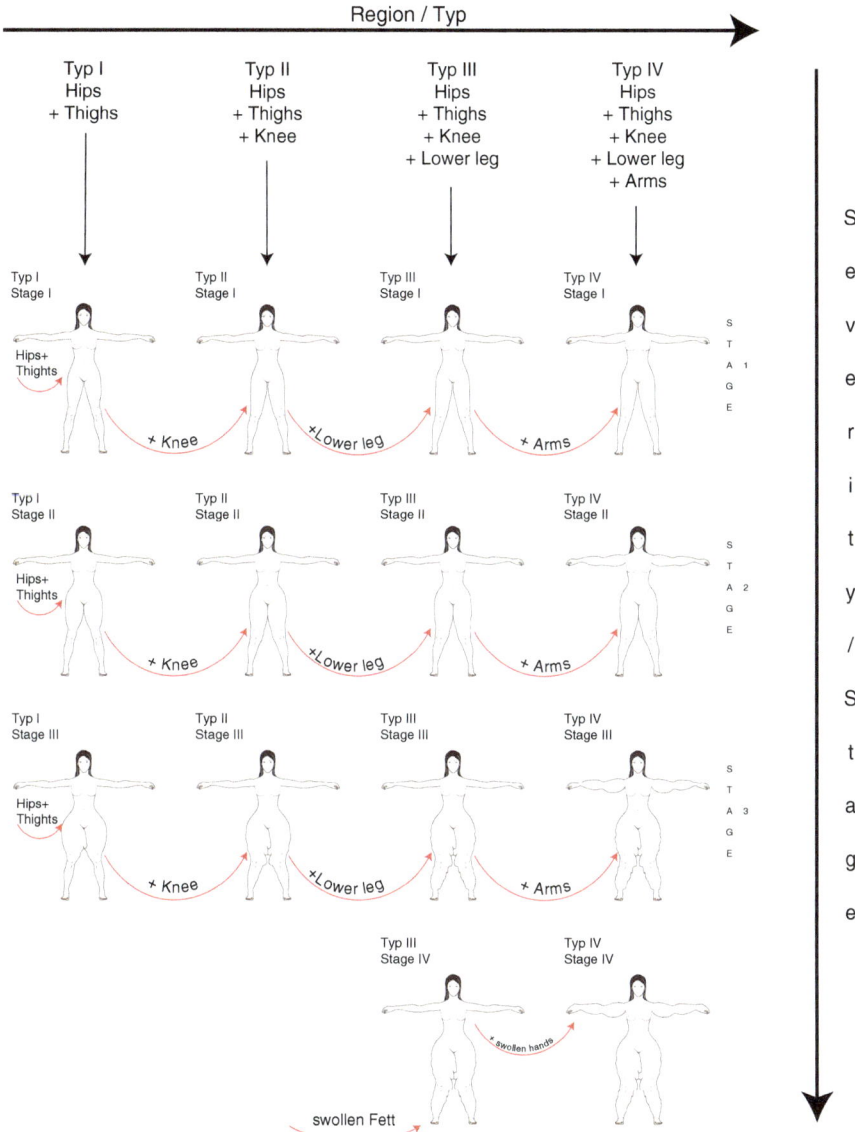

Fig. 1.32 Type and stage classification at a glance

"Stage 1: Smooth skin surface with uniformly thickened, homogeneously imposing subcutis.

Stage 2: Uneven, predominantly wavy skin surface, nodular structures in the thickened subcutaneous area.

Stage 3: Pronounced circumferential proliferation with overhanging portions of tissue (dewlap formation)."

Speaking from our experience, which forms of lipedema we see most often in our consultation, we can note the following gradations.

1. Combination of obesity and lipedema with lipedema of the hips and thighs.
2. Normal weight or slightly overweight affected persons with lipedema in the area of the hips, upper and lower legs, plus arms if necessary.
3. Normal weight or slightly overweight affected person with a columnar leg, plus arms if necessary.
4. Normal weight or slightly overweight affected individuals with buttocks, hips, upper and lower legs, plus arms if necessary.

Many people ask us if there is also lipedema on the abdomen, face, and back. Typically, lipedema does not occur on the back, abdomen, and face. However, if we define lipedema as a painful fat distribution disorder, then in principle it can occur anywhere on the body. We count painful fat, outside the regions of hips, arms and legs as atypical lipedema. Many colleagues do not consider lipedema of the buttocks as lipedema. We see it differently. The buttock region is certainly a region that is often painfully affected and forms a unit especially with the hip and upper thigh region.

▶   By atypical lipedema, we mean lipedema that is not visible at first glance or painful adipose tissue in atypical regions. The term "atypical lipedema" has been coined by us.

We would like to comment on the current type and stage classification.

As we have already noted, the type and stage classification is merely descriptive. Neither the intensity of pain nor the extent of movement restriction nor the psychological burden (manifest mental illness excluded) is taken into account.

Unfortunately, in Germany, the staging is used to establish a medical justification for surgical therapy. This is a major problem. It is also difficult that in this classification a stage applies to the entire body. However, it may be that the disease progression in the area of the thighs corresponds to a stage III, but in the area of the lower legs to a stage II or vice versa.

So, we see that the classification is not quite as simple as it seems at first glance. As with many other diseases, lipedema is not only black and white but also gray, sometimes even light gray and dark gray.

It is precisely this gray area that represents a major challenge in the treatment of lipedema. The many intermediate and special forms must be given appropriate individual consideration in therapy. It would therefore make more sense to use a classification that takes more account of the pathological changes.

In an effort to improve all these, we have developed our own classification. In addition to the classic types already described, there are buttock-only, hip-only, thigh-only, and lower leg-only types. Even though in our daily clinical routine these are rather rare, we see affected persons who only have complaints in the upper or lower arms or the whole arm. Therefore, we distinguish each individual body region from one another in our classification (Fig. 1.33). Depending on the affected region, a simple type code can be created. This means that we can always see exactly which regions are affected.

By combining the numbers and letters, it is then possible to clearly determine exactly which regions are affected by lipedema. If, for example, both legs are completely affected and both upper arms are affected, we speak of type VI/A, which is actually quite simple and straightforward. This classification makes it possible to combine very many variations of the affected areas.

In our opinion, the current classification of stages also needs to be revised. There are indeed women who have strong or more severe symptoms in the early stages of

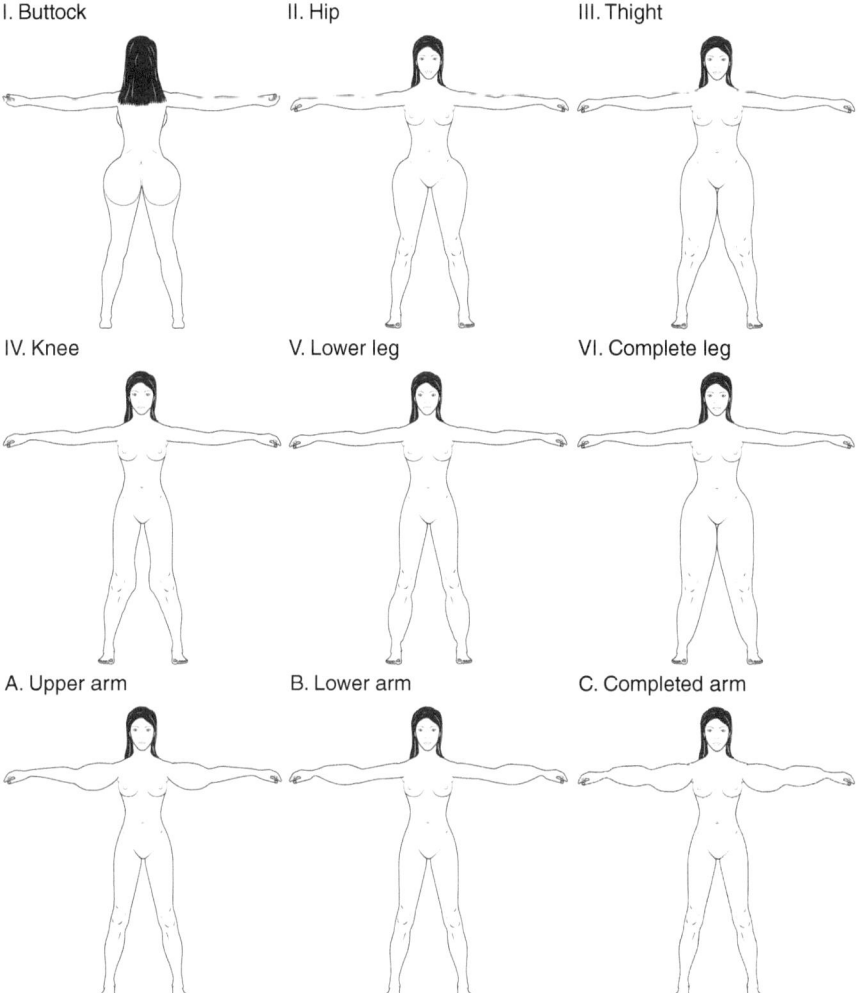

Fig. 1.33 New, individual type classification

lipedema than other patients in a higher stage. Unfortunately, this fact is not taken into account in the current staging, which severely limits its validity.

▶ The current type and stage classification should be revised.

In addition, the staging is spongy and not concrete enough. The transitions between the stages leave too much room for discussion.

Therefore, we postulate not only a new type of classification but also a new stage classification, which we collect using a 21-page questionnaire tailored to lipedema and an associated score system. This results in a concrete diagnosis and stage of all affected regions. However, even our staging is only as good as the main symptom of the disease, pain, can be objectively assessed. Despite questionnaires, this is extremely difficult. The pain (P = pain) is then indicated using the score of 0–10 per region. We will go into more detail on establishing the diagnosis in Sect. 1.9.

The stage also includes the regional manifestation of lipedema or lipohypertrophy. For this purpose, we use a scale from + to +++ depending on the severity for the respective region. Furthermore, our staging classification indicates the extent of edema (E = edema) and restriction of movement (D = disability), each with a value of 0–4 (Table 1.9). This staging is hardly suitable for everyday use, but it is recommended for medical documentation and better analysis of lipedema.

Lipedema of the hip/thigh and lower leg and arms could be classified as follows: II +/P3/E0/D0—III +++/P8/E0/D1—IV ++/P0/E0/D0 − A +/P2/E0/D0. The interpretation is presented in Table 1.10.

Table 1.9 New, individual stage classification

Symptom	Abbreviation	Scale
Regional severity	–	+ to +++
Intensity of pain	P (pain)	1–10
Extent of edema	E (edema)	1–4
Extent of movement restriction	D (disability)	1–4

Table 1.10 Example classification of lipedema in the hip/thigh, lower leg, and arm area

Classification	Regional manifestation	Pain P	Edema E	Movement restriction D
II +/P3/E0/D0	Hip Little pronounced	Level 3 (lipedema, since >0)	No edema	None
III +++/P8/E0/D1	Upper leg Strongly pronounced	Level 8 (lipedema, since >0)	No edema	Little
IV ++/P0/E0/D0	Lower leg Moderately pronounced	None (no lipedema, since 0)	No edema	None
A +/P2/E0/D0	Arms Little pronounced	Level 2 (lipedema, since >0)	No edema	None

In this way, each region can be described in detail. For the sake of simplicity, we will continue to use the classic classification of lipedema in the remainder of the book.

Another fundamental aspect that needs to be discussed is the naming of the disease. The name "lipedema" is unfortunately only partially appropriate for the clinical picture, as it is always associated with the presence of edema, which is not true in most cases.

The word "edema" often quickly establishes a close relationship to lymphedema. However, this is a completely different and independent clinical picture with no relationship to lipedema. The conclusion derived from this that lipedema is treated like lymphedema is also incorrect. The rare case of lipo-lymphoedema must be considered separately.

The call for a new name is not new and is also advocated by other experts in this field. Let's take a look at our neighboring countries and see what they have to say on the subject:

This is how our colleagues in the United Kingdom view the issue in their guidelines, "The management of lipoedema" (https://www.lipoedema.co.uk/):

Lipoedema is predominantly a chronic adipose tissue disorder (the word lipoedema means 'fat swelling'), with clinically apparent oedema due to fluid accumulation in the tissues occurring as a secondary feature in some individuals (Todd, 2010; Herbst, 2012a; Reich-Schupke et al, 2013; Herbst et al, 2015). Although most commonly called lipoedema, the condition has a variety of other names.

Meaningfully translated, this means:

Lipedema is predominantly a chronic adipose tissue disorder (the word lipedema means "fat swelling"), with clinically apparent edema in the sense of fluid accumulation in the tissues occurring as a secondary feature in some individuals (Todd, 2010; Herbst, 2012a; Reich-Schupke et al, 2013; Herbst et al, 2015). Although the condition is most commonly referred to as lipedema, it has a number of other names.

The Lipedema Guidelines in the Netherlands can be found on the Internet at the following address: https://nvdv.nl/. We take the liberty of reprinting this text passage:

A major obstacle is the limited available scientific literature, along with inconsistency concerning the diagnosis of lipedema. The condition is characterized by symmetrical accumulation of fat tissue with typical clinical characteristics, generally in the extremities (more detail provided later). Lipedema is an unfortunate term, as it often evokes the idea of swelling due to fluid accumulation. However, it refers to swelling—in the sense of an increase in volume—due to increased fat tissue.

Meaningfully translated, this means:

A major problem in lipedema is the poor scientific situation in terms of literature and inconsistencies in diagnosis. The condition is characterized by a symmetrical accumulation of adipose tissue with typical clinical features, preferably in the extremities (more details later). Lipedema is an unfortunate term because it often evokes the idea of swelling due to fluid accumulation. However, it is a swelling—in the sense of an increase in volume—due to increased adipose tissue.

Table 1.11 Classification of adipose tissue diseases

Form	Type
Painful type	Lipalgia or lipodolorosa (chronica)
Movement-restricting types without pain	Functional fat distribution disorder
Painless type	Lipohypertrophy/fat distribution disorder

▶   Conclusion: Lipedema should not be called lipedema, but rather adipose tissue disease.

Lipedema is simply a fat disease. This group of fat diseases should then be subdivided into subcategories, each of which has its own disease value (Table 1.11). Lipo-lymphedema would not be affected by this and would remain as such.

1.9   Diagnosis

By a diagnosis, we understand the determination and naming of a disease. In the diagnosis phase, we work toward establishing and naming the disease.

▶   By a diagnosis we mean the identification and naming of a disease.

With lipedema, the phase of diagnosis can be comparatively quite long. At least this is true for many lipedema sufferers we see in our practice and tell their story of suffering. Often it is because those affected do not know where and to whom they should present themselves. In addition, many colleagues are not familiar with the clinical picture and in many cases make an incorrect diagnosis or no diagnosis at all.

Diagnostic Criteria
As we have already indicated in Sect. 1.8, lipedema has a decisive disadvantage compared with other diseases: there are no objectifiable diagnostic criteria for lipedema. This means that no examination is available with which lipedema can be detected with certainty. There is neither an objective imaging nor an objective laboratory value nor an objective fine tissue examination (examination of a tissue sample) nor any other objective parameter that can undoubtedly diagnose lipedema.

In this context, we speak of so-called soft and hard parameters. Soft parameters, in contrast to objective parameters, are criteria that can be interpreted in different ways. The soft parameters thus offer a large scope for discussion.

For a better understanding of this issue, the following examples may help:

1. You stumble and fall on your right hand. Because you are in pain and your hand is also swollen, you consult a doctor. In this case, an X-ray of your right hand is taken for diagnostic purposes. If the X-ray shows a fracture, it is certain that the bone is broken. There is no need to discuss this.

2. You suffer from shortness of breath and visit your family doctor, who will arrange various examinations. An ultrasound examination could then reveal, for example, that you are suffering from cardiac insufficiency. This also leaves rather little room for discussion.

In both examples, the diagnosis is confirmed by an objective procedure that cannot be challenged.

The situation is different with lipedema, where the objective criteria are completely lacking. This is a major problem—a problem of traceability, a problem of recognition, a problem of billing, and a problem of differentiation from other diseases. But the problem is not just objective diagnosability. Rather, the difficulties begin with understanding the disease. To date, we know very little about the causes, development, or reasons for the development and progression of lipedema. A therapeutic approach aimed at curing the disease therefore simply does not exist.

Due to the fact that these objective diagnostic criteria do not exist, there can also be no exact figures in terms of frequency and new occurrence of the disease. The figures that sometimes appear in the press are only rough estimates.

Very often we experience in our clinical everyday life that lipedema is misdiagnosed. On the one hand, this means that a diagnosed lipedema is not present in the affected person at all, or that an actual lipedema is not recognized as such. This is usually difficult for sufferers of both situations to understand. If we can confirm the diagnosis, we often see enormous relief in the patients. It is worse when we have to say that it may not be lipedema after all.

In general, the earlier a diagnosis is made, the sooner treatment can be initiated. So if you think you suffer from lipedema, you should see an "expert." How to find such a specialist, you will read in the further course.

The path to diagnosis can vary greatly from physician to physician. In our practice, in front of a case of suspected lipedema, we proceed by collecting

1. the medical history (anamnesis) of the person concerned. This step is followed by,
2. an observation (inspection) of the affected parts of the body and,
3. a physical examination (palpation).

In all three parts of this protocol, there are typical constellations that speak for or against lipedema. The procedure is supported and recorded by a questionnaire.

Medical History

To begin with, we ask you what is the driving force behind your introduction to us. The answers to this question turn out to be very diverse. For many of those affected, the feeling of fear of suffering from a fat distribution disorder is at the forefront because they have noticed changes in shape that are atypical for themselves. Others have had chronic, almost unbearable pain for years. The range is really very wide. Classically, those affected report that a visible fat distribution disorder has already set in with the onset of puberty. For many, this is still painless at that time, for others it is already painful.

▶   A fat distribution disorder/lipedema usually begins with puberty.

Of particular interest to us is exactly which areas are affected. Here, too, there are definitely differences. While some complain of complaints in the legs only, others report pain in the legs and arms. For others, only the hip–buttock region is affected, or even a completely different region of the body.

A relapsing course of the disease is often described. However, this is not always the case. We also see, for example, older patients in an initial stage in which they have been for several years without observing any progression. Very typical are relapses in phases of hormonal change. This also fits the theory of hormonal dependence. These include puberty, pregnancy, and the onset of menopause.

Furthermore, it is interesting for us to know whether your mother, grandmother, or other relatives have or had similar complaints. It is not uncommon for a fat distribution disorder to be inherited.

Even if you have already described your complaints to us in detail, we will usually ask you a few more questions. Not because we have not listened to you, but because there are some core questions that are essential for our and your diagnosis. Some of these questions revolve around the pain issue. Namely, if there is a painless fat distribution disorder, then by definition we are talking about simple lipohypertrophy. If it is lipohypertrophy with pain, then by definition it is lipedema. It is therefore not a myth that lipohypertrophy is distinguished from lipedema solely by the presence of pain.

The pain itself is usually described as rather nonspecific. However, both the quality and intensity of the pain are known to exhibit a wide range. This is exactly why we have our lipedema questionnaire.

▶   Our lipedema survey form can be downloaded at http://www.lipold.de.

Sample questions include: What type of pain is present? Pressure pain, tension pain, touch pain, or tearing pain? Does the pain tend to occur at rest or with exertion? Does the pain increase during the day? Is there also pain at rest?

The pain symptomatology plays a major role for us, as the type and intensity of the pain often indicate certain other diseases that should be ruled out—even if lipedema is suspected.

▶   By definition, a painless fat distribution disorder is not lipedema and is referred to as lipohypertrophy.

In addition, regular feedback on the success of each treatment is important for us to be able to constantly adapt and improve it. The questioning of pain before and after an operation thus also serves our own quality assurance.

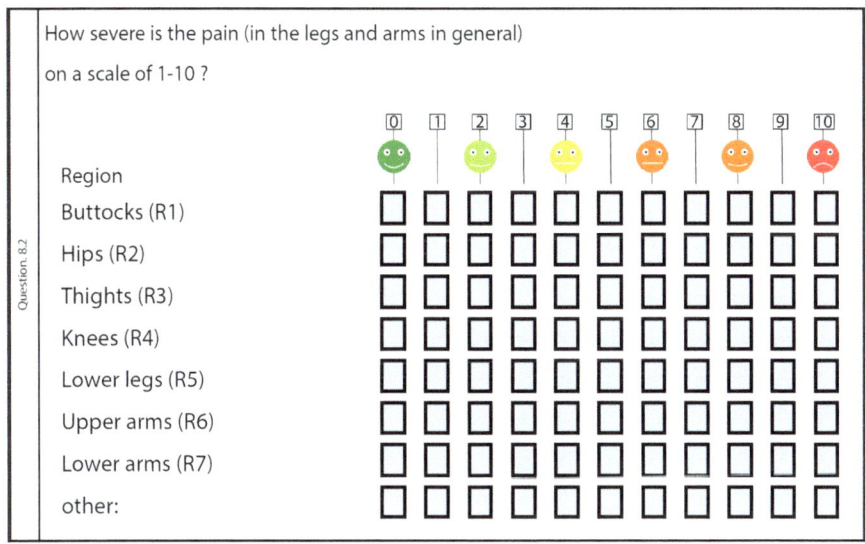

Fig. 1.34 Example question from our lipedema survey questionnaire

To record pain, we use a so-called visual analog scale in our questionnaire (Fig. 1.34). The visual analog scale (VAS is used to record subjective attitudes, in this case, pain.

However, the VAS can also be recorded in practice, for example, using a pain slider or in writing. In the written version, a horizontal bar is usually given, on which a cross is placed according to the extent of the sensation queried. Either we ask explicitly for a pain value (0 = no pain, 10 = strongest pain) or we use the template.

With the stencil, the rating is done on the scale from one extreme (far left) to the opposite extreme (far right). Often equipped with a slider, this can be slid over the printed numbers from 0 to 10.

However, not only the intensity and quality of the pain play a role for us. The question of the duration of the pain is also relevant for us. From a period of about 6 months, we speak of chronic pain. Whereby the period for "chronic" is defined somewhat differently and generally lies between 3 and 12 months. Ultimately, the decisive factor for our treatment strategy is to weigh up whether pain or dissatisfaction with the external appearance is the main issue. Filtering this out is, as you can imagine, a balancing act.

In addition to pain, we are also interested in any kind of disturbed sensibility in the affected parts of the body. Is there a strong sensitivity to touch? For example, do you have a feeling of tension or heaviness in your legs or arms?

What about bruises? Do you bruise quickly? Although bruising in lipedema is controversial, we raise this symptom as a possible indication of lipedema.

What about water retention in the sense of edema? When do you observe this phenomenon and how does it behave during the course of the day? Does it improve or worsen during the day? How it responds to which treatment?

We also ask about subjective physical limitations. To what extent is there a restriction of movement and thus a reduced performance capacity that prevents you from mastering your everyday life without complaints? Do you experience restrictions at work? What about sports?

Finally, to get a good overall view of the history of the disease, we also ask how satisfied you are with your body image, what stresses you experience as a result of this and how you deal with your situation. In the further conversation, we also go into your course of the disease and your previous therapy.

Inspection

Now that we have talked in detail about the entire complaints, your examination follows. During the examination, we determine to what extent we can objectively understand the fat distribution disorder described by you. It is important to look at the entire body, including the arms, hands, feet, and the entire torso area. It is important not to look at the affected regions in isolation, but to form a relationship between the different regions.

In the case of a combination of fat distribution disorder and obesity, it is necessary to determine exactly which disorder is the main problem. This is crucial for the therapeutic approach. To objectify this relationship, there are parameters that help us. We will discuss these later in this section.

But how obvious or how disproportionate does a fat distribution disorder have to be for us to speak of lipedema? Can lipedema still be in the foreground if obesity is pronounced, or should perhaps the obesity be treated first?

These key issues, along with pain symptomatology, are the central questions that need to be answered in terms of the best possible treatment.

▶ Lipohypertrophy/fat distribution disorder in favor of the extremities is a relatively sure sign of lipedema if pain symptoms are present at the same time.

Difficult to assess is atypical lipedema, especially borderline cases, at both ends of the extremes. For example, there are patients in whom lipedema is ruled out because it is not outwardly obvious or is only very mild, but the patients nevertheless suffer from lipedema. The same applies to very obese patients in whom the accompanying obesity may rule out lipedema from the outset for the inexperienced observer. This is a very unsatisfactory situation for both groups. Here it is necessary to make the correct diagnosis with a great deal of tact and experience.

▶ There are forms of lipedema that exist WITHOUT an obvious fat distribution disorder, especially in very slim affected individuals.

Another element we need to pay attention to is the skin. Questions we need to ask ourselves here are: What is the skin texture? Have flaps of skin already formed? Sometimes we see a so-called collar- or muff formation on arms and legs. This phenomenon describes an abrupt jump in caliber from the affected to the unaffected area, which then causes the external appearance of a collar or muff (Fig. 1.35).

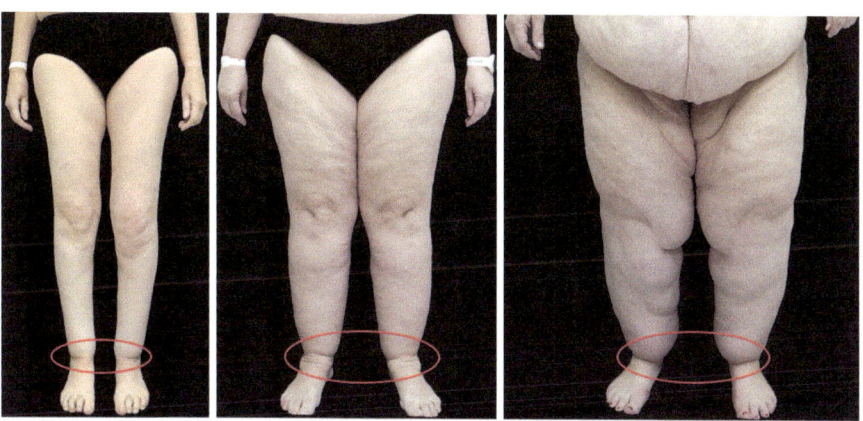

Fig. 1.35 Collar formation at the transition between the lower leg and foot with different degrees of lipedema

But beware. Skin-soft tissue excess, as defined for stage III, can also occur in patients after massive weight loss. We see a significant number of patients after gastric bypass and massive weight loss in which the clinical appearance resembles stage III lipedema, although there was never any discomfort or disproportionate fat distribution disorder.

Palpation Examination
This is followed by a physical examination. Softness and turgor of the tissue? Is palpation painful?

To check for the presence of edema, we first examine the pressure-related behavior of the tissue. We distinguish between edema that can be pushed away and edema that cannot be pushed away (the name "pushable" is unfamiliar, but it is the correct term for it). Edema that can be pushed away responds to pressure. Usually, this pressure is applied by the thumb or another finger during the examination. If the skin of an area of edema is depressed with the thumb, a "dent" or depression will remain even after the thumb is removed. This takes some time (longer than 2–3 s) to level out to skin level again. In the early stages, edema can usually be pushed away, whereas in the advanced stages it cannot be pushed away due to the associated tissue changes and thus no "dent" remains in the tissue (Fig. 1.36).

After checking the impressionability, we examine the hands and feet. The aim here is to determine whether the backs of the feet and/or hands are also affected. The so-called Stemmer's sign gives us a clue. To do this, an attempt is made with the index finger and thumb to lift a fold of skin over the second or third toe or the dorsum of the foot. If an edema component is present, no skin fold can be lifted off and the Stemmer's sign is positive (Fig. 1.37). If no edema component is present, then a skin fold can be lifted off and Stemmer's sign is negative. If Stemmer's sign is positive and a fold cannot be lifted off the dorsum of the foot, there is certainly NO pure lipedema. It could be lymphedema, lipo-lymphedema, or edema of a different etiology.

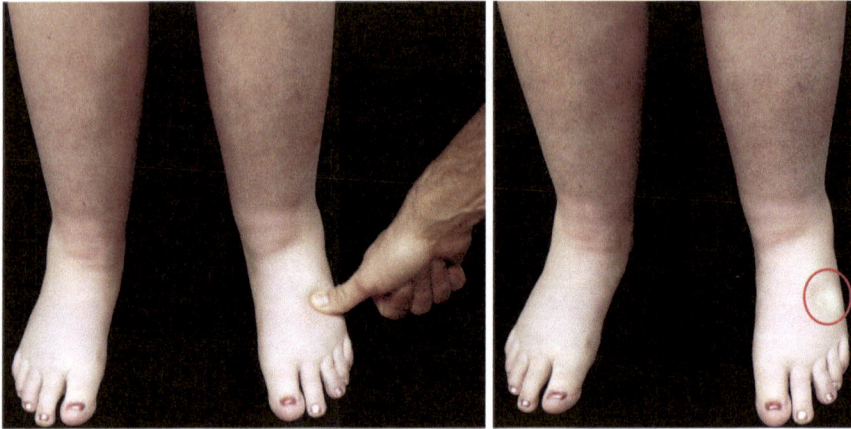

Fig. 1.36 Edema test by indentation

Fig. 1.37 Edema test by attempting to lift off a skin fold (Stemmer positive)

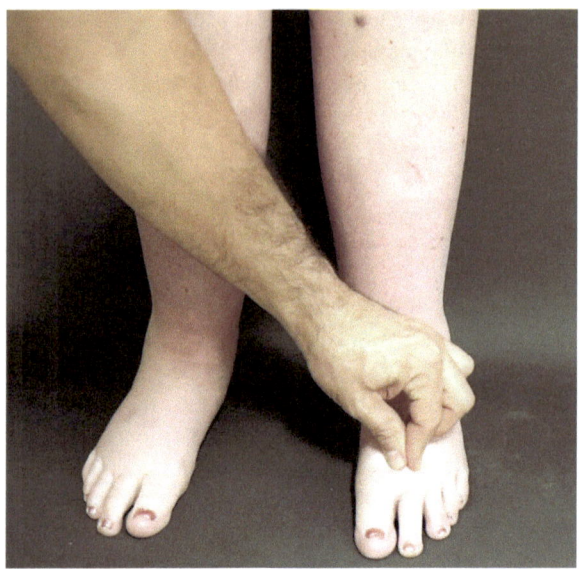

To examine the painfulness, we can use the so-called pinch test. It should be said in advance that the test is widely used but not very specific. It merely tests the extent to which there is increased sensitivity to pain in the affected areas. For this purpose, a healthy and supposedly diseased area is pinched at the same time. The pinching is performed with moderate force. In the case of lipedema, those affected usually feel more pain in the diseased area than in the healthy area.

▶ The pinch test is not very specific.

When evaluating this examination method, it must be noted that this is a purely subjective test procedure. Here again, we encounter the problem that the subjective perception of pain offers no possibility of objectifiability. Despite the limited evaluability, the test can serve as another piece to complete the puzzle.

Imaging Diagnostics

As we have already stated, there are no apparative diagnostics that either prove or exclude lipedema with certainty. Since other conditions besides lipedema and lymphedema can be associated with swelling of the legs or arms, we may send you to other specialists to have certain tests performed. It is important to rule out other conditions in advance or, if necessary, to treat them. One example is chronic venous insufficiency, a vein disease that can cause edema of the legs even in its early stages. So, in the case of swollen legs, an evaluation by a phlebologist, angiologist or vascular surgeon is often recommended as well. Often, an ultrasound examination is then performed to examine the vessels.

▶   To rule out other causes for the symptoms, a presentation to a phlebologist, angiologist, or vascular surgeon should be made.

An ultrasound examination can also be used to measure skin thickness. Many colleagues speak of a "thicker" skin in lipedema, which can be detected by ultrasound. In a 2018 study by Hirsch et al. (Halle, Germany), there were no differences regarding skin thickness in lipedema patients compared to healthy or obese individuals. However, a thickening of the skin is often seen in lymphedema patients, so that a skin layer thickness measurement can be useful in these patients.

Others speak of larger fat cells on ultrasound. However, there is no evidence for this, especially when comparing lipedema areas with those of purely obese people.

Even though we use a high-resolution ultrasound machine on a daily basis to plan other surgical procedures, we do not see any additional benefits of using an ultrasound machine in lipedema diagnosis.

To further differentiate between lipedema and lymphedema, we sometimes perform an infrared camera imaging of the lymphatic vessels, which in borderline cases, provides us with decisive information about the cause of the swelling. For this purpose, we inject a dye in the area of the interdigital or interfinger furrow. After a waiting period of a few minutes, we use a special infrared camera to view superficial lymphatic vessels and how they transport the dye away. While the examination works very well in the early stages of lipedema, we are limited in advanced stages. This is because this method can only visualize very superficial lymphatic vessels. Since we do not usually see concomitant lymphedema in lipedema, we do not regularly use this examination method for this purpose.

Continuing imaging studies such as lymphoscintigraphy and lymphangio-MRI also do not provide any benefit in the diagnosis of lipedema.

Diagnosis

Let us now turn to how we consolidate and finalize our diagnosis. We have gathered a lot of information in the conversation and during the examination and now want to substantiate this with objective data. As we already know, this is not always easy.

Especially in the case of a fat distribution disorder or lipedema, in which subjective factors largely determine the symptoms, we must try to find objective factors and criteria that help us make a diagnosis. Also, with the knowledge that these factors are not an expression of the actual pain intensity, movement restriction, and restriction of the quality of life and that there is the atypical lipedema.

In terms of body weight, we roughly distinguish five groups (with many transitional stages), so-called body shapes (Fig. 1.38).

The five body shapes for the affected people with lipohypertrophy or lipedema are

– Underweight.
– normal body weight,
– slightly increased body weight,
– strongly increased body weight and,
– extremely overweight.

Affected persons who are underweight are basically not seen at all. Each of these groups must be treated differently—not fundamentally differently but in a graduated manner (see Sect. 3.4, The individual therapy plan).

We already talked about the BMI (body mass index) for the classification of obesity in Sect. 1.3. Unfortunately, the BMI only takes into account pure weight as well as the pure height and does not do justice to different body compositions. For example, athletes with a lot of muscle mass and little fat can have an increased BMI value, just like obese people.

If we look at the number of lipedema sufferers in the group of the severely and extremely obese, we can roughly say: the higher the body weight, the more sufferers of lipohypertrophy and lipedema are found in these groups. This supports the thesis that in the case of a multifactorial genesis of lipedema (i.e., it is triggered by various causes) obesity is one of the causes.

A large group of lipedema sufferers are not overweight per se, although they are led to believe so by an increased BMI. This happens when the fat distribution disorder is very pronounced. Therefore, it is enormously important in these sufferers that we do not use BMI alone or even BMI at all to assess lipedema.

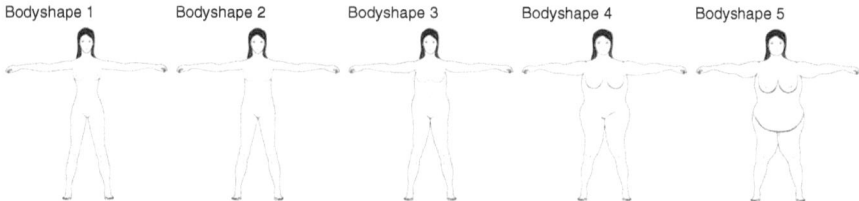

Fig. 1.38 Five different body shapes

BMI is a parameter/index for evaluating body weight in relation to height, nothing more.

▶   BMI, body mass index or also called body measurement index, is an index for evaluating body weight in relation to body size.

$$\text{BMI} = \frac{m[kg]}{l^2[m^2]}$$

The BMI is given in the unit of measurement kg/m². The body mass m is divided by the body height l2, where m, the body mass, is given in kilograms and l, the body height, is given in meters.

However, the BMI helps to get a rough orientation: rather normal weight, rather slight overweight, rather strong overweight. This can certainly be derived from the BMI. If you have a present, clearly visible fat distribution disorder with pain in these regions, a tendency to bruise and a BMI of up to 34 kg/m2, the presence of lipedema is more likely than not. However, if you suffer from a significant fat distribution disorder, you should not use the BMI value as a reference. This will then not apply to you. There are other values that can be consulted instead of BMI. These include:

1. waist–hip ratio (WHR),
2. waist-to-height ratio (WHtR).
3. circumference and volume measurements of the extremities.

Thereby, to get a quick impression, the Waist–Hip Ratio and Waist-to-Height-Ratio are interesting.

Waist–Hip Ratio
The Waist–Hip Ratio (WHR) relates the circumference of the waist to the circumference of the hips. The number, that is, the ratio, is given as a simple number without a dimension or unit.

To obtain the waist–hip ratio, the smallest waist circumference (centrally between the lowest rib and the upper edge of the pelvis) and the hip circumference in the area of the largest circumference are measured in a standing position with the arms resting against the body (Fig. 1.39).

$$\text{WHR} = \frac{u[m] = \text{waist circumference}}{l[m] = \text{hip circumference}}$$

For example, the waist-to-hip ratio for a waist circumference of 80 cm and a hip circumference of 100 cm = 0.8.

$$\text{WHR} = \frac{T\text{waist}(80\,cm)}{\text{hip}(100\,cm)} = 0,8$$

Fig. 1.39 Waist–hip ratio

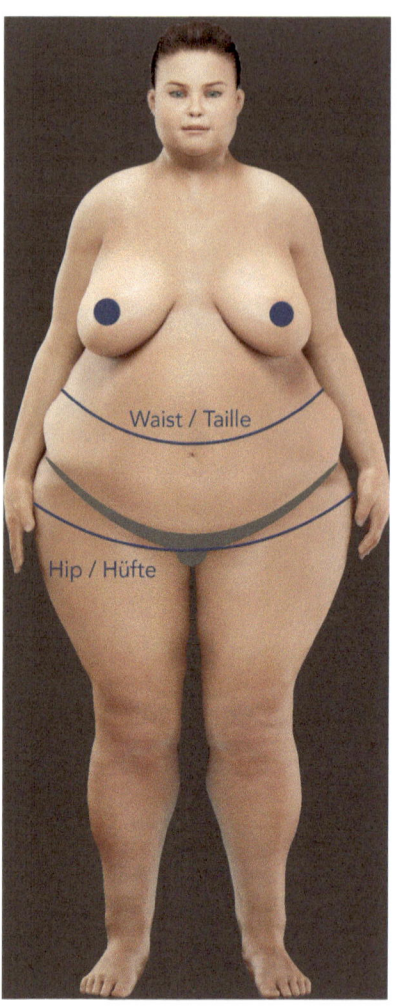

Normal values are considered to be a WHR <0.9 in men and <0.8 in women. Obesity is defined from a WHR of >0.85 in women and >1.0 in men. The situation is different when there is a disproportion, as in lipedema, in favor of the hips. The more pronounced the disproportion, the smaller the WHR.

$$\text{WHR} = \frac{Twaist\,(80\,cm)}{hip\,(130\,cm)} = 0{,}69$$

▶ The greater the disproportion between the waist and hips, the smaller the waist-to-hip ratio.

Thus, the WHR can be used to assess forms of lipohypertrophy or lipedema that are particularly localized around the hips and buttocks. Thus, if one has an increased BMI but a small WHR, this should be taken as a sign of disproportion.

Waist-to-Height Ratio (WHtR)

The waist-to-height ratio is another tool for assessing the severity of lipedema or lipohypertrophy. This measure is particularly suitable for assessing body fat distribution in affected individuals who have a marked fat distribution disorder without underlying obesity (Table 1.12). It is also suitable for assessing health risks.

$$WHtR = \frac{u[m] = \text{waist}}{l[m] = \text{height}}$$

$$WHtR = \frac{\text{waist}\,(80\,\text{cm})}{\text{height}\,(170\,\text{cm})} = 0,47$$

Example in lipedema patients:

$$WHtR = \frac{\text{waist}\,(90\,\text{cm})}{\text{height}\,(170\,\text{cm})} = 0,53$$

▶ If there is a disproportion as in lipedema in favor of the hips with a normal waist, a WHtR should be in the normal range. Even if the BMI should be high and the WHtR is in the normal range, this speaks for a fat distribution disorder and not for obesity.

Circumference and Volume Measurement of the Extremities

A circumference and volume measurement can also be useful, especially to record a progression. When measuring the circumference, we recommend measuring the hips, waist, torso alongside the inframammary line, at the very top of the upper arm, in the middle of the upper arm, at the level of the crook of the elbow and in the area of the middle forearm, at wrist level and the circumference of the hand when the hand is stretched out flat. On the leg, analogously, in the area of the thigh close to the body, at mid-height, at knee height, in the area of the lower leg close to the body, at ankle height, and in the area of the middle foot. There are also standard tables with marked locations where the measurements should be taken. We have our own protocol for these values, which has become established over the years. In Fig. 1.40 you can see the measurement regions. Of course, both arms and legs must be measured.

There are also volume measurements, for example, with the aid of modern 3D cameras, via water displacement, and many more, which would go beyond the scope of this article.

Table 1.12 Reference values of the WHtR

Age	Critical range
< 40	>0,5
40–50	0,5–0,6
>50	>0,6

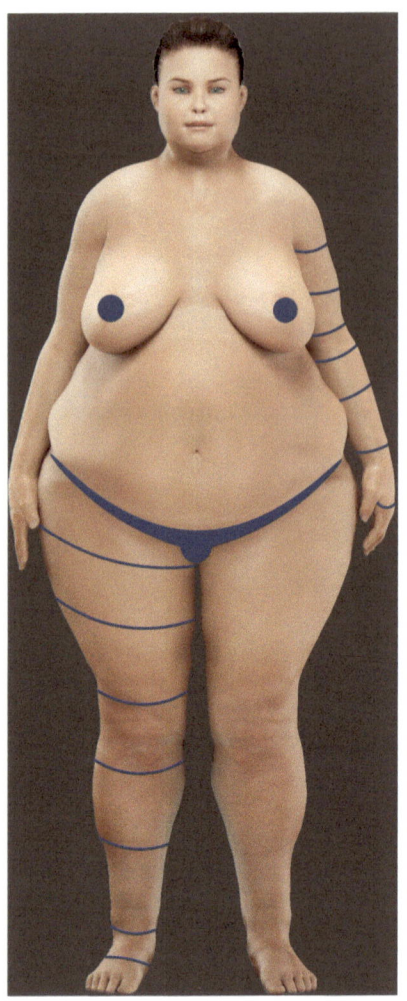

Fig. 1.40 Circumference measurement on arms and legs

From all the data collected above, the interview, the examination, the palpation findings, the data on BMI, WHR, and WHtR, we finally derive the diagnosis.

If you were to ask us what we would like to see in the future, it would be simpler and better diagnostics. But what could better diagnostics look like? If it were possible, for example, to send a sample of subcutaneous fat tissue or even a blood sample to a laboratory and detect lipedema via a test, that would be perfect. What would be the consequences if such objective diagnostics were possible? The health insurance companies would certainly reevaluate the disease and cover the costs of treatment due to the reliable diagnosability.

What needs to be done until then? We have to work with the tools at our disposal, support science, and try to establish standards.

The Lymphedema

2

Corrado Campisi, Lucian Jiga, and Zaher Jandali

In this chapter, we will look at both the similarities, but mainly the differences between lipedema and lymphedema.

The differences result from the different causes of both diseases. These differences are not always clear to the layperson and are often difficult to understand due to the medically complex interrelationships. It should become clear that, despite some similarities, these are two completely different clinical pictures, which differ significantly from each other in their development, symptoms, diagnosis, and therapy.

However, notwithstanding these differences, the problem is up to now under discussion, and related research is in progress, considering moreover the potentially compromising lymphatic drainage in dysfunctional adipose tissue and the possible, even if relatively rare, evolution of the initial pure lipedema to the lipo-lymphedema state, depending, of course, on lipedema worsening staging.

2.1 Anatomy and Functioning of the Lymphatic System

Our body has two vital transport systems. In addition to our blood circulation, which transports oxygen from the lungs to the tissues and carbon dioxide back, supplies our cells with nutrients and acts as a transport route for hormones, components of blood clotting, and defense, there is a second, almost parallel transport route in our body. This is the so-called lymphatic system (syn. Lymphatic system). While the

C. Campisi (✉)
Adjunct Professor University of Catania. Plastic, Reconstructive and Aesthetic Surgery, Lymphatic Surgery and Microsurgery, Private Consultant Genoa, Milan, Rapallo, Reggio Emilia, Genova, Italy
e-mail: corrado.campisi@campisiandpartners.com

L. Jiga · Z. Jandali
Department of Plastic, Aesthetic, Reconstructive and Hand Surgery, Evangelical Hospital Oldenburg, Oldenburg, Niedersachsen, Germany
e-mail: dr@jandali.de

© Springer Nature Switzerland AG 2022
Z. Jandali et al. (eds.), *Lipedema*, https://doi.org/10.1007/978-3-030-86717-1_2

function and structure of the blood circulation are usually well known, the lymphatic system is far less familiar to most people. In the following, we want to change that and give you an understanding of the basic features of the lymphatic system.

As already mentioned, the lymphatic system is also a transport system of our body. On the one hand, it serves to remove fluid from the tissues and thus keep the fluid balance in equilibrium, and on the other hand, it serves as a means of transport for so-called lymphatic substances. These include proteins, fats, bacteria, viruses, and foreign bodies that cannot be absorbed by the capillaries of the blood vessels due to their size. Our lymphatic system is therefore often disparagingly referred to as the "body's garbage disposal system." In addition, the lymphatic system has an indispensable task in immune defense.

To fulfill all these tasks, this unique and highly specialized organ system of our body has a very special structure (Fig. 2.1). On the one hand, it consists of the lymphatic vascular system, on the other hand of the lymphatic organs. The latter, in turn, can be divided into primary and secondary lymphatic organs.

The primary lymphoid organs are responsible for the formation and maturation of progenitor cells into mature immune cells. These include the thymus and bone marrow. The secondary lymphoid organs are where the contact between the mature immune cells and antigens takes place. In addition to the lymph nodes, they include special tissues in the gastrointestinal tract (mucosa-associated lymphoid tissue), the pharynx (pharyngeal, palatine, and lingual tonsils), and the spleen.

Primary Lymphatic Organs

The primary lymphatic organs include the bone marrow, which is located inside all bones, and the thymus, a small gland located in the upper mediastinum. This is where the formation and maturation of special defense cells called lymphocytes or "white blood cells" takes place. The formation of all lymphocytes begins in the bone marrow. Depending on whether their maturation into functional defense cells also takes place in the bone marrow or the thymus gland, a distinction is made between B ("bone marrow") and T ("thymus") lymphocytes. B and T lymphocytes fulfill various tasks of the body's defense system. These include the production of antibodies or the recognition and destruction of viruses or degenerated cells (e.g., cancer cells).

Secondary Lymphatic Organs

Secondary lymphoid organs include the spleen, lymph nodes (Fig. 2.2), and mucosa-associated lymphoid tissue. In these tissues, the so-called antigen presentation and recognition take place. In a sense, the lymphocytes are taught here against which antigens they have to act and how.

The lymphatic vascular system begins with the initial lymphatic vessels, often referred to as lymphatic capillaries or lymphatic collectors. They are the smallest sections and begin as a network between the capillaries of the blood circulation in the intercellular space of organs or the skin. The diameter of such a lymphatic capillary is about 50 µm, which is about 10 times larger than that of a blood capillary. Their task is to absorb tissue fluid and dissolved substances. From here, the lymph

Fig. 2.1 Structure of the
lymphatic system

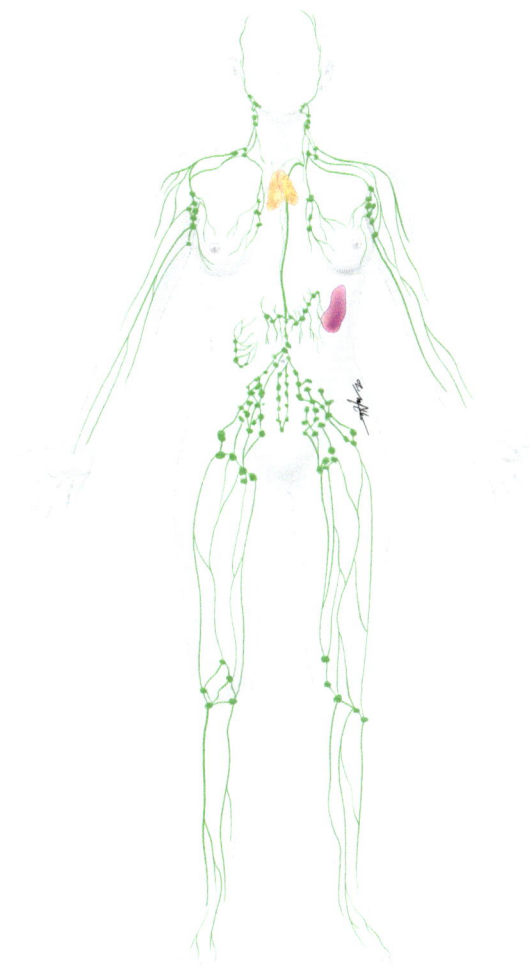

is transported to the larger lymphatic vessels. They are formed by the union of several lymphatic capillaries into so-called precollectors. Several lymph nodes are interposed in these and basically serve as a filtering station. A special feature of the lymphatic vessels is the many interposed valves that facilitate the transport of the lymph and prevent backflow (Fig. 2.3).

Several lymphatic vessels then unite to form the lymphatic trunks, which are usually arranged in pairs. In these lymph trunks, the lymph fluid is collected in each case from a specific region of the body. From here, it is drained into the left and right vein angles via the lymphatic ducts, which form the last section of the lymphatic pathway, and is thus fed into the bloodstream. With the exception of the lymphatic vessels that drain lymph from the right arm and right head and neck region, all lymphatic vessels converge into the main lymphatic trunk (thoracic duct). This eventually drains into the left subclavian vein. Lymph vessels from the right arm and the

Fig. 2.2 Cross section of
a lymph node

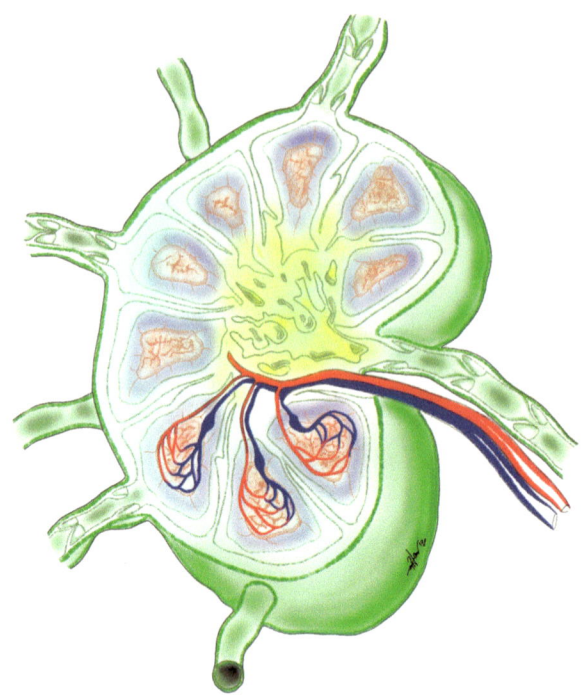

Fig. 2.3 Cross section of
a lymphatic valve

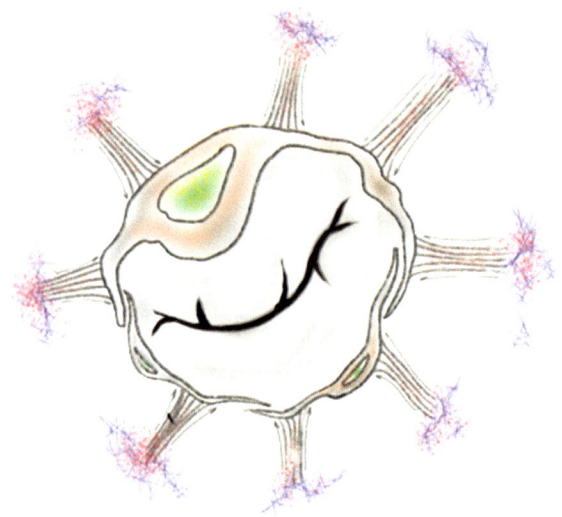

right head and neck region, on the other hand, drain into the right lymphatic duct (Ductus lymphaticus dexter), which in turn ends in the right subclavian vein.

Due to this special architecture, the lymphatic system essentially fulfills three different tasks.

Firstly, it acts as a transport system. Every day, approx. 2–3 L of the ultrafiltrated interstitial fluid is reintroduced into the bloodstream. The transport takes place on the one hand passively by contraction of the surrounding skeletal muscles, and on the other hand actively by a peristaltic movement of the muscles built into parts of the lymphatic vessels. The interposed valves prevent the lymph from flowing back (Fig. 2.3).

Secondly, the lymphatic vascular system fulfills an important function in the body's defense system. Through the intermediate lymph nodes, pathogens that can easily penetrate the lymphatic vascular system due to the high permeability of the lymphatic capillaries can be freed. Furthermore, the lymphatic vascular system serves as a transport medium for lymphocytes.

Thirdly, it is the task of the lymphatic vascular system to absorb or transport lipids (fats). Glycerol and fatty acids are absorbed via special lymphatic vessels of the gastrointestinal tract, the so-called chyle vessels, which also have a very high permeability. This allows lipids to be supplied directly to adipose tissue and muscle without first passing through the liver. Due to the high fat content after passage through the digestive tract, the lymph changes its appearance here from clear to milky turbid. In addition to the high fat content, the lymph contains numerous plasma proteins, coagulation factors, and fibrinogen, as well as cellular components (mainly lymphocytes).

Interestingly, the central nervous system is left out of the lymphatic system to protect the brain. This extends from the outside only as far as the meninges. However, there is an indirect connection to the lymphatic system via the brain's own disposal system.

2.2 Causes

Lymphedema is a complex clinical condition. Approximately 140–250 million people worldwide suffer from it. It is caused by a lack of transport capacity of the lymphatic system, which means that the interstitial fluid (tissue fluid between the cells) can no longer be adequately removed, resulting in a backlog of lymph in the intercellular spaces. This appears as a visible and palpable accumulation of fluid, which is accompanied by fibrosis of the tissue (the connective tissue loses its functional properties) and excessive storage of fatty tissue, especially in advanced stages. The lower and upper extremities are most frequently affected. Based on the cause, primary (congenital) is distinguished from secondary (acquired) lymphedema.

Primary Lymphedema/Congenital Lymphedema
Primary lymphedema, which describes the rarer form of lymphedema, is a congenital disorder of the lymphatic vascular system or the lymph nodes, which are either not formed at all or are formed incorrectly.

▶ In primary lymphedema, the lymphatic vascular system is congenitally disturbed.

Most often, there is hypoplasia (lack of formation) of the lymphatic vascular system or a reduced number of lymphatic vessels in a particular region of the body. The lymphatic drainage of the lower extremity is most frequently affected. Less commonly, valvular disorders may also occur. Primary lymphedema occurs sporadically in about 97% of cases and is therefore not inherited. The primary form usually manifests itself with the onset of puberty and can occur unilaterally or bilaterally. Women are affected about twice as often as men.

Secondary Lymphedema/Acquired Lymphedema

This is an acquired damage of the lymphatic system, as a result of which there is a disturbed outflow of the lymph.

▶ Secondary lymphedema is caused by acquired damage to the lymphatic system.

Common causes are accidents, tumor diseases or inflammation of the lymphatic vessels, chronic venous insufficiency (chronic venous congestion), and diabetes mellitus. The most common cause worldwide is lymphatic filariasis, an infectious disease caused by the so-called nematode (*Wuchereria Bancrofti*). In our latitudes, however, this disease plays a minor role. Mostly it is caused by treatments such as surgery, radiation, or the removal of lymph nodes in the course of tumor surgery. The most common example of this is probably secondary lymphedema of the upper extremity (arms) after lymphonodectomy (removal of lymph nodes) from the axilla in breast cancer (Fig. 2.4).

The risk of developing lymphedema of the arm ranges from 9 to 41% in cases of radical lymph node removal and 4–10% in cases where only the sentinel lymph node was removed. Somewhat insidious is the usually delayed onset of lymphedema after surgery; several months to years often elapse. In breast cancer-associated lymphedema, the first symptoms appear on average 8 months after axillary dissection (lymph node removal from the axilla), 75% during the first 3 years. Once onset, the subsequent course of secondary lymphedema is usually highly variable. Some patients may experience only mild, painless, and nonprogressive swelling that does not require therapy, while others may experience rapid progression associated with a severe reduction in quality of life. Unfortunately, if left untreated, the progressive course is the rule rather than the exception.

▶ The incidence for the occurrence of lymphedema of the arm ranges from 9 to 41% in cases of radical lymph node removal and 4–10% in cases where only the sentinel lymph node was removed.

The same applies to the lower extremity as to the upper extremity. Lymphedema can also occur in the head and neck or genital area after lymph node removal. Thus, lymphedema is not limited to the extremities. In addition, there are many reports

Fig. 2.4 Lymphedema in
the area of the left arm
after breast cancer

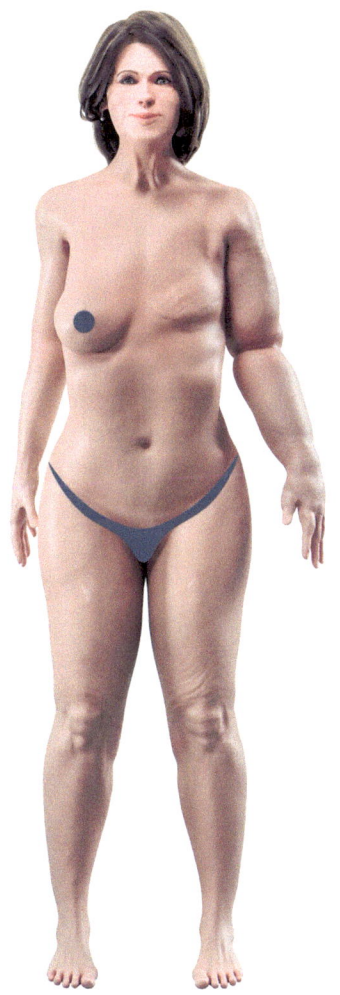

from EBM literature confirming that also secondary lymphedemas related to lymph node removal, often recognize congenital dysfunctional and/or dysplastic latent impairments of the underlined loco-regional lymphatic system.

Malignant lymphedema is a subgroup of secondary lymphedema. In this case, either progressive tumor grows itself or metastasis leads to obstruction of the lymphatic vessels.

2.3   Clinical Appearance

Depending on its expression and classification, lymphedema can be divided, according to the updated ISL Consensus Document, into three different stages (modified by Campisi Staging, 2009), each of which is accompanied by a more or less characteristic appearance.

In the latency stage (stage 0), no symptoms appear yet. It is characterized by reversible, subthreshold edema.

In stage I, a visible and palpable doughy-soft swelling can already be detected. However, this can usually be reversed spontaneously by elevation. Smaller fibrosclerotic tissue changes (changes from functional tissue to connective tissue with a resulting loss of function) may occur in isolated cases.

Stage II is already characterized by marked fibrosclerotic changes and the proliferation of fatty tissue. The palpation changes from formerly doughy-soft to rather hard. At this stage, elevation no longer leads to spontaneous regression. Whereas in stage I, it is still easy to "press in" a dent in the edema area, this is hardly possible in stage II.

Stage III shows the maximum expression of lymphedema. Extensive fibrosclerotic changes and often massive fatty tissue proliferation are evident, which severely restrict natural movement. As edema progresses, the skin tends to develop eczema, erysipelas, or vesicles. Symptomatically, pain, feelings of tension, and a characteristic feeling of heaviness of the affected body part usually occur in the early stages (Fig. 2.5).

2.4   Diagnosis

The medical history is of decisive importance and the first step in the basic diagnosis of lymphedema. Past operations, past infections, tumor diseases as well as vascular diseases or skin changes that may have seemed insignificant up to now, in combination with the corresponding symptoms, already provide initial indications of the presence of lymphedema. A positive family history can also be a further clue.

Furthermore, the assessment of the clinical appearance is elementary, because the external examination can provide information at an early stage as to whether the complaints described are lymphedema or not. In this context, attention is paid to the localization of the swelling and any differences in circumference, which can be just as decisive as the assessment of the skin in terms of color, skin changes, temperature, and texture.

The third decisive step in the initial lymphedema diagnosis is the palpation findings. This is similar to the examination in lipedema. We also check the Stemmer's sign here. It is considered a reliable feature for detecting the presence of lymphedema. However, some caution is required here. A negative Stemmer's sign does not necessarily rule out lymphedema. Palpation also includes the assessment of lymph nodes with their size, consistency, displaceability, and tenderness. Palpation also checks for edema consistency and reliability.

▶   A negative Stemmer's sign does not rule out lymphedema.

To confirm the diagnosis and to discuss the extent and location of the damage to the lymphatic system in more detail, various other diagnostic procedures can help.

Fig. 2.5 Stage III
lymphedema in the left leg
after pelvic lymph node
removal

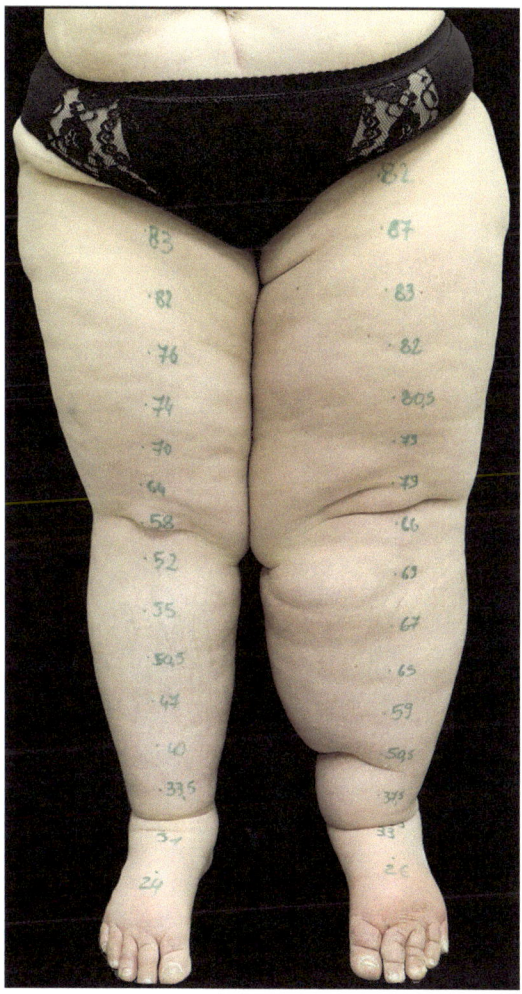

Among the imaging procedures, we distinguish morphological from functional diagnostics. Sonography, MRI, and indirect lymphangiography provide information about morphology. Function can be assessed by functional lymph scintigraphy (Campisi et al. 2019; Villa et al. 2019) and fluorescence microlymphography. Indocyanine green lymphangiography (ICG) is also increasingly used.

We perform an apparative diagnosis by means of an indocyanine green lymphangiography. A liquid, fluorescent dye is injected into the patient's skin. This is absorbed by the lymphatic vessels and transported away (Fig. 2.6). The figure shows the cloudy dye injection site in the area between the toes and the good removal of the lymph via the well-illustrated, linear superficial–subdermal lymphatic vessels. The fluorescent dye can be seen and assessed via an infrared camera connected to a monitor (Figs. 2.7 and 2.8) (Campisi et al. 2018; 2020).

Fig. 2.6 ICG

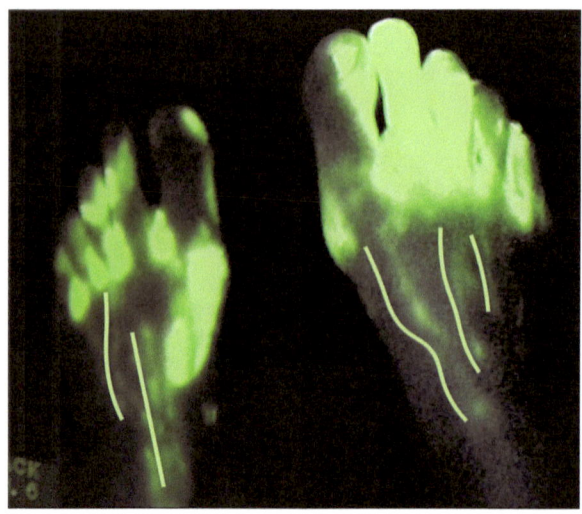

2.5   Conservative Therapy

Lymphedema is a chronic and usually progressive disease that requires long-term treatment (Fig. 2.9). Therapy includes both conservative and surgical measures and aims to prevent the progression of the disease and alleviate existing symptoms.

Before recommending any therapy, we conduct a medical history survey. Likewise, each patient is thoroughly examined and any additional diagnostics are also performed. Together with the results of the medical history, diagnostics, and examination, we are able to offer patients a treatment plan that is individually tailored to their condition.

The basis of conservative lymphedema therapy is based on a combination therapy of manual lymphatic drainage (MLD), compression therapy, movement exercises, and skin care developed as early as the 1970s. The complex therapy consisting of these four components is summarized under the term "Complex Physical Decongestive Therapy" (CPD). CPD is considered the gold standard and the first-choice therapy for lymphedema.

▶   CPD (complex physical decongestive therapy) is considered the gold standard and the therapy of the first choice.

Manual Lymphatic Drainage
Manual lymphatic drainage (MLD)is a special form of physiotherapeutic treatment in which the removal of lymph is promoted with targeted hand movements. On the one hand, the accumulation of fluid from the interstitium toward the lymph capillaries is supported in this way, and on the other hand, the self-transport within the lymph vessels is stimulated, which favors the removal of further lymph.

Fig. 2.7 Lymphedema in
the area of the arm

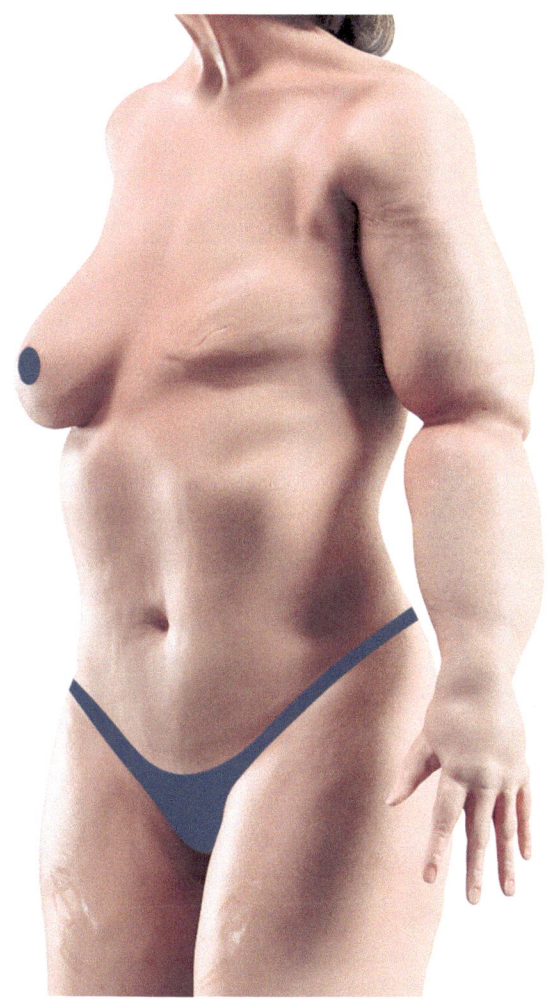

In addition to manual lymphatic drainage, appliance-based lymphatic drainage can be performed. Special devices can perform lymphatic drainage at home via an adapted peristaltic compression cuff. There are different providers here, although the devices work according to the same principle. These devices are available from the relevant providers via a prescription after requesting cost coverage from the health insurance company.

Compression Therapy
Compression therapy is also an important component of CPD. The affected part of the body is wrapped with bandages. The pressure applied from the outside supports the drainage of the lymph, and the pressure decreases toward the trunk to ensure a directed lymph flow. For lymphedema, we recommend flat-knit compression garments made to measure, including the hands and feet.

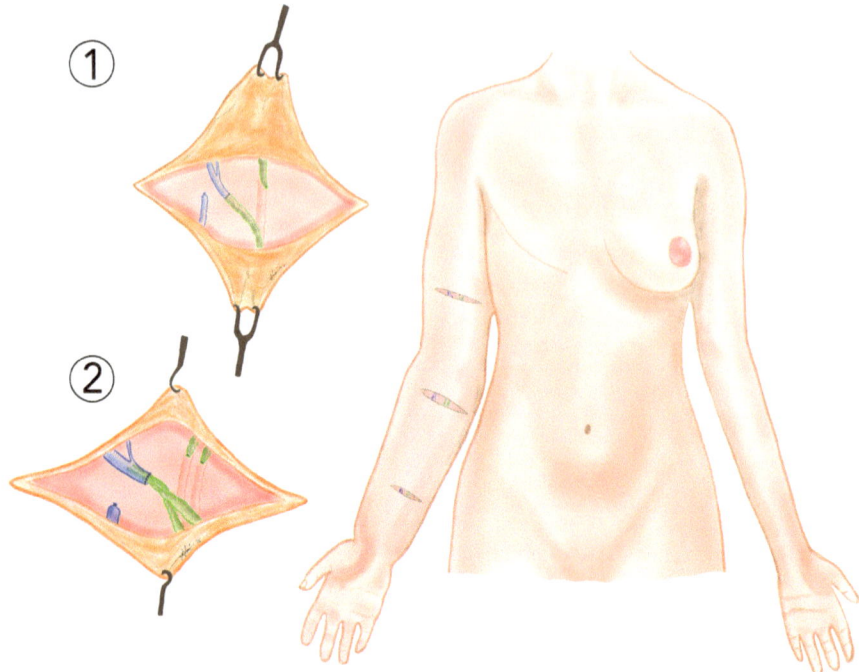

Fig. 2.8 Lymphovenous (1) and multiple lymphovenous anastomosis (2)

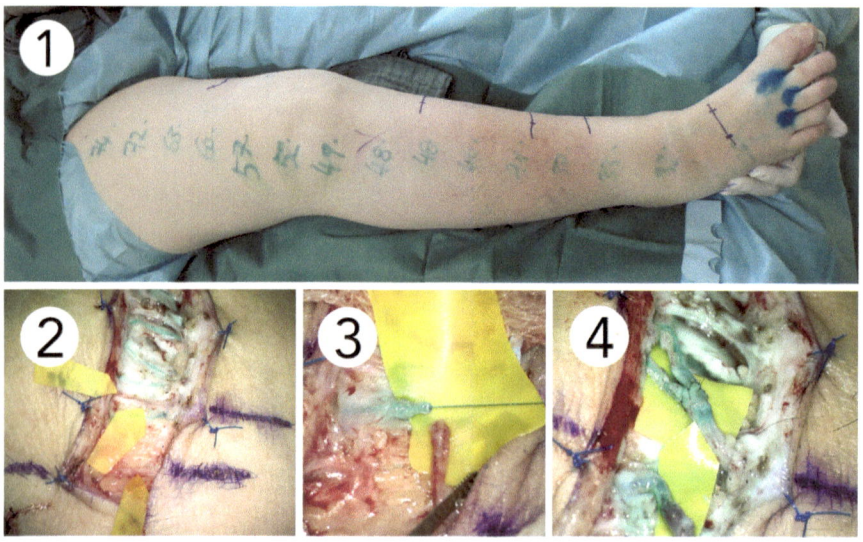

Fig. 2.9 Clinical images of planning and relocation of lymphatic vessels

Movement Exercises

Targeted movement exercises are designed to increase lymph drainage. Among other things, the natural activation of the muscle pump thus promotes passive lymph transport. It is important that an individually tailored therapy program be developed for each affected person.

A new advanced specific protocol is under assessment, in Genoa, named BioCircuit, with tailored exercises by an exclusive Computer Assisted Technology.

Skin Care

Daily skin care is an indispensable pillar of CPD for lymphedema patients. Due to the usually compromised natural skin barrier, the skin is significantly more susceptible to infections. Especially via furrows and rhagades (smallest tears in the skin) germs can penetrate the body and cause severe infections. Bacteria have an easy time spreading due to the defective lymphatic system and poor metabolism in the region.

▶   For those affected by lymphedema, skin care is essential to prevent serious infections.

CPD is divided into two phases. In the first, so-called decongestion phase, the existing edema is to be reduced as much as possible. In this stage, daily treatments are carried out by means of manual lymphatic drainage, compression therapy by means of wrapping, movement exercises, and skin care. The bandage is worn continuously, except during treatment. Depending on the stage, this phase can last several weeks.

Once the edema has been reduced as much as possible, the maintenance phase begins. The main purpose of this second phase is to maintain or improve the results already achieved. At the beginning of this phase, a flat-knitted compression stocking is fitted. Unlike the circular knitted stocking, this stocking is not stretchable in all directions and therefore provides better compression. In the maintenance phase, the therapy concept also consists of manual lymphatic drainage, compression treatment, movement exercises, and skin care. However, lymphatic drainage usually, in the earliest stages (IB, IIA), no longer has to be performed daily, but from 3 to 4 times a week to 1–2 times every 14 days, depending on the extent. Wrapping, in these cases, is also now only done on the day of therapy. On any other day, the compression stocking can be worn. Often, the initial treatment takes place within the framework of a rehabilitation measure in a clinic specialized for this purpose.

2.6   Surgical Therapy

To understand the therapy of lymphedema, it must be noted that lymphedema is often a chronically progressive disease. It is associated primarily with the sometimes massive accumulation of lymphatic fluid, fibrosclerotic tissue changes, massive fat tissue proliferation, and ultimately also the destruction of lymphatic pathways.

As described above, each patient receives an individual therapy plan. Although often, in advanced stages (IIB, IIIA, and IIIB), a long-term treatment for lymphedema/elephantiasis, CPD has established itself as the gold standard in therapy. The prerequisites for the success of this cure are lifelong implementation and strong compliance on the part of each patient.

If CPD does not achieve the desired success, various surgical options are available in addition to conservative therapy, with the goal of preventing the progression of edema, reducing excessive volume, and improving the aesthetics and function of the affected region.

In principle, a distinction is made between two different approaches. On the one hand, there is the restoration (reconstruction) of lymphatic drainage. This can be achieved, for example, by means of lympho-lymphatic bypasses, lympho-venous anastomoses, performed as lymphatico-venular superficial scattered microanastomoses or as single-site multiple deep and superficial lymphatic-venous anastomoses, or with the so-called vascularized lymph node transfer. Yes, you are right: this sounds complicated, but we will explain these complicated terms in a moment. In contrast, there are resecting (= tissue-removing) procedures that aim purely to reduce mass or volume. These include liposuction and excision (simply cutting away) of the diseased tissue.

Let us first discuss the reconstructive options for lymphedema treatment. In these surgical measures, we distinguish techniques,

– based on surgical treatment of the lymphatic vessels,
– transplant the lymph nodes, and,
– which aim to resprout lymphatic vessels.

2.6.1 Restorative/Reconstructive Surgery

Advances in the field of surgery have now made it possible to identify microscopic lymphatic vessels and assess their quality during surgery. This opens up the possibility of at least partially restoring impaired lymphatic drainage. We would like to explain various techniques to you below.

Lympholymphatic Bypass
This technique can be used, in selected cases, to bridge individual sections with restricted lymphatic drainage. For this purpose, an endogenous lymphatic vessel (or vein) is removed from a region of the body not affected by lymphatic drainage. This lymphatic vessel is then connected to functional sections of the lymphatic vessel system both far from the body and close to the body of the drainage disturbance. The lower the stage of lymphedema, the more promising this technique is. Individual studies have demonstrated up to 80% reduction in the circumference of the affected limb. A disadvantage is that in isolated cases lymphedema may occur in the region of the removed lymphatic vessel.

Lymphovenous Anastomoses

These methods represent today the most frequent microsurgical techniques applied in clinical practice for lymphedema treatment.

A direct connection between the lymphatic system and venous circulation is also established here. The advantage over lymphovenous bypass is that the removal of a donor vessel can be dispensed with. In fact, with this technique, lymphatic vessels are connected to smaller veins in the immediate vicinity. Individual studies describe a subjective improvement in symptoms in up to 95% of patients after such an intervention. The great advantage of this scar-saving technique is the comparatively less traumatic procedure, which significantly reduces the perioperative risk. In isolated cases, wound healing disorders or the formation of lymphatic fistulas may occur.

The figure (Fig. 2.11) schematically shows a (1) lymphovenous anastomosis (LVA) and (2) multiple lymphovenous anastomosis (MLVA). The difference between LVA and MLVA is that in MLVA, a single lymphatic vessel is not connected 1:1 with a vein, but several lymphatic vessels are inverted into a vein and connected. In Campisi's experience single-site MLVA is performed at the inguinal crural region for lower limb lymphedema, and at third medium-superior of the volar surface of the arm for upper limb lymphedema. In addition, Campisi does not use a cross skin incision along the limb, except to approach the inguinal crural region.

Figure 2.9 shows a lymphedema patient in our operating room. Images 2–4 were taken with 50x microscope magnification. Lymphatic vessels were visualized via injection of indocyanine green (1). Subsequently, the lymphatic vessels and veins were visualized. The yellow plastic arrows point to the veins, and the blue–green colored vessels are the lymphatic vessels that absorbed the dye from the tissue (2). For a lymphatic vessel to be sutured, we (Jandali–Jigas's Technique) cannulate it with a hair-thin thread (3). In picture (4) the completed detour of the lymphatic vessels into veins can be seen.

Vascularized Lymph Node Transplantation

One of the newer techniques of lymphedema therapy is free vascularized lymph node transfer (Fig. 2.10). The principle is the removal of a lymph node package, including its vascularization, from an unaffected part of the patient's own body and the transplantation of this package into the area of lymphedema. In theory, two different mechanisms triggered by this procedure are thought to improve lymphatic drainage. Firstly, the transplanted lymph nodes act as a kind of sponge, so to speak, sucking up the lymph in the region and directing it toward the lymphatic vessel. On the other hand, the lymph node transplantation results in a new lymph vessel sprouting in the area surrounding the lymph node. The newly formed lymphatic vessels then carry the lymph to the lymph node, and from there, further, metabolization occurs via the vein of the lymph node into the venous circulation. Several body regions can be used as donor sites. The groin region, the chin, and neck area or the area above the collarbone and lymph nodes from the abdominal cavity have become established. We most frequently remove lymph nodes from the abdomen, as the risk of suffering lymphedema as a result of the removal is significantly reduced in this area.

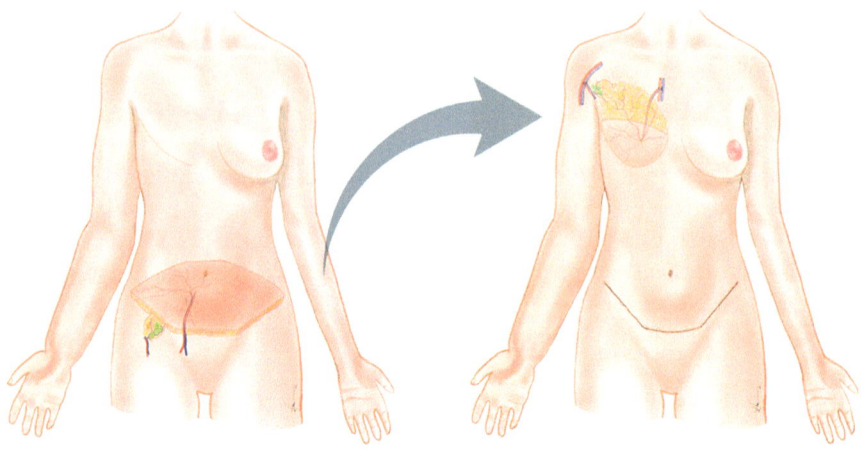

Fig. 2.10 Clinical images of planning and relocation of lymphatic vessels

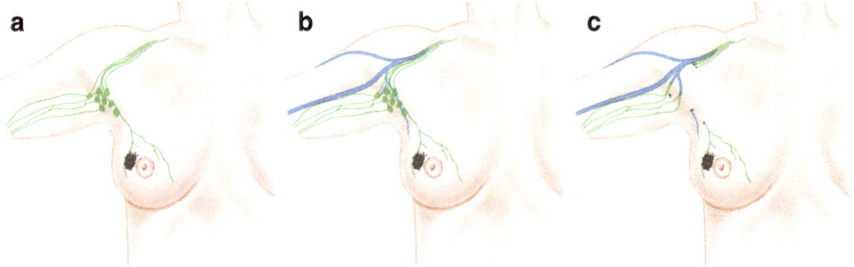

Fig. 2.11 The LYMPHA principle

However, research is in progress to establish the potential risk of malignant degeneration in the transfer site, reported in some recent articles, due to the growth factors locally induced by lymph node transfer on the immune altered lymphedematous tissue, with lymphangiosarcoma (like Stewart–Treves Syndrome) or carcinoma frightful implant. That is why, on the ethical, deontological, and medicolegal points of view, this terrific event, even if exceptional, would be considered and clearly explained to the patient, acquiring his/her informed consensus.

Das LYMPHA-Prinzip (Lymphatic Microsurgery Preventive Healing Approach)

An example of lymphedema treatment that we perform very frequently is the combined treatment of breast reconstruction after breast removal and lymphedema treatment after lymph node removal from the armpit. For breast reconstruction, the transfer of excess skin-fat tissue from the abdomen is performed. In addition, a lymph node package is relocated from the groin to the armpit. Finally, the removed tissue is connected to the local blood supply in the recipient area.

Due to the anatomy of the upper extremity lymphatic drainage, lymphedema often develops on the arm of the affected side after breast removal in combination with lymph node removal. The removal of multiple lymph nodes in combination with the injury to multiple lymph vessels from surgery can be compensated for to some degree, but are also eventually exhausted.

Due to the progress in the field of microsurgery in the course of the last years, it is nowadays possible for us to identify these damaged lymphatic vessels and to restore them immediately. On the one hand, this can be done by directly suturing the injured lymph vessels or by connecting the lymph vessel to a vein in the surrounding area.

In practical terms, this means that a trained plastic surgeon joins the operation during the lymph node removal from the armpit and diverts the injured lymph vessels directly into veins (i.e., as a precaution). This extends the total operation time by 30 min and requires good cooperation between oncological and plastic surgery teams. Studies have shown that this significantly reduces the risk of lymphedema.

In Fig. 2.11, we show the principle of LYMPHA operation. (A) Before tumor removal. The dark dot above the nipple represents the tumor, green the lymphatic vessels. (B) As (A), but with veins. (C) After tumor and lymph node removal and redirection of lymph vessels into draining veins.

2.6.2 Tissue Removal Measures

Liposuction
We will discuss liposuction in detail in Chap. 3, Treatment of lipedema. Its primary purpose is to reduce the increase in subcutaneous fatty tissue observed in advanced lymphedema. Although it primarily leads to a reduction in circumference and an associated improvement in function and aesthetics of the affected limb, studies also show a marked improvement in lymphatic drainage after surgery. There appear to be several explanations for this: First, tissue injury during surgery could result in connections between lymphatic vessels and veins, allowing lymph to be delivered directly to the bloodstream. On the other hand, injuries to the respective muscle fasciae could promote drainage of the lymph from the superficial to the deep lymphatic vascular system, which actually makes more sense.

In summary, liposuction for the treatment of lymphedema is a comparatively low-risk procedure, only if performed by lymph vessel sparing procedure, on the guide of the fluorescent ICG microlymphography. In this way, the risk of aggravating lymphedema during surgery by injuring remaining, functional lymphatic vessels is quite low if the technique is correctly adopted. On the contrary, if liposuction is performed without this kind of lymph vessel procedure, due to the total lymph vessel debulking, the consequent heavy charge is the permanent and mandatorily need to continue wearing compression garments for the rest of the patient's life. Then, debulking blind liposuction is not a measure that restores lymphatic drainage, and therefore is more likely to be noted as a fallback option. In Campisi's experience, as a matter of fact, lymph vessel sparing selective liposuction (by this author preferably named fibro-lipo-lymph-aspiration, to avoid any possible confusion with the blind liposuction) is regularly performed as a sequential complementary therapeutic procedure, after MLVA microsurgery, for the effective treatment of advanced lymphedema.

In any case, plastic surgeons today have to be very careful in applying liposuction, even if for only aesthetic indications, and have to be skilled to respect lymph vessels during this procedure.

Overall, the pre- and postoperative care, as well as the surgical procedure, differs from liposuction for lipedema. For example, before surgery, the edema must be minimized as best as possible. Likewise, compression must be worn much more consistently after surgery.

To be updated on this topic concerning relationships between lymphatics and lipedema, both on theoretic and on practical points of view, it is mandatory to explain that, although assuming the specific differences between lipedema, lymphedema, and the relatively rare lipo-lymphedema, there are recent review articles in which is underlined that "expanding adipocytes produce some lymphangiogenic factors, such as VEGFC, which may induce lymphatic hyperplasia. Lastly, in hypoxic environments, hypoxia-inducible factor 1 enhances fibrosis, thus potentially compromising lymphatic drainage in dysfunctional adipose tissue. Taking into account these findings, research is still needed to clarify whether a persistent and progressive damage of the microlymphatic vessels because of adipose tissue expansion, rather than a primary lymphatic defect, may be responsible for the lipo-lymphedema state" (Buso, Mazzolai et al., Obesity, 2019: 27, 10, 1567–1576).

In Campisi's recent experience there is an exemplary case of a lipedema, initially diagnosed by other specialists as a pure lipedema, in which superficial and deep lymphoscintigraphy, according to the Genoa protocol (with the additional calculation of the transport index), showed a latent functional and clinical impairment of the lymphatic circulation, allowing us to perform the proper tailored treatment by MLVA at the inguinal crural region.

To conclude, approaching lipedema surgery, the skilled plastic surgeon must be sure that the lymphatic system is functionally intact and, in any case, it has to be respected during the surgical procedure.

Tissue Removal/Debridement (Charles Procedure)
Radical removal of the areas affected by lymphedema (skin and subcutaneous tissue) is nowadays reserved exclusively for the most severe forms of lymphedema. The aim of this technique is to remove the skin with all underlying fatty tissue down to the respective muscle skin and then cover it with a skin graft. However, the improved function of this procedure is offset by the unsightly result and the high surgical risk (Fig. 2.12).

If it were now a matter of explaining how we make our decision as to when to use which procedure, it would go a little too far. If surgical reconstruction is indicated,

Fig. 2.12 Principle of the
Charles operation

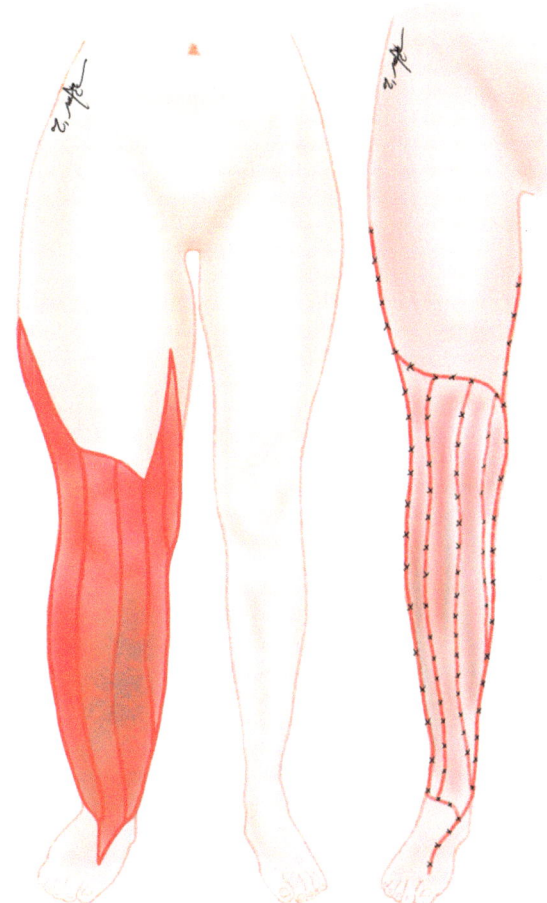

we make our decision based on the individual lymphatic vessel status and the overall medical history. Currently, according to Jandali's procedure, lymph node transplants are most frequently performed, followed by lymphovenous "shorts", obtaining better results with lymph node transplantation than with lymphovenous detour. In Jandali's experience, the majority of cases (except for lymphedema following axillary lymph node removal after breast cancer), is treated by harvesting lymph node packages from the gastric region. The removal is performed laparoscopically through only three small incisions. The subsequent transplantation usually takes place quite quickly within 2–4 h.

According to Campisi's experience, the majority of cases is treated by MLVA (alone, in the stages I A-B and II A), and followed by sequential fibro-lipo-lymphaspiration with lymph vessel sparing procedure for stages II B, III A–B.

2.7 Similarities and Differences of Lipedema and Lymphedema

It is not uncommon for lipedema to be referred to as lymphedema or other diseases or to be confused with them. As explained in detail in the previous sections, these are fundamentally different clinical pictures whose causes, diagnostic possibilities, and therapies largely differ greatly from one another.

Gender Distribution
Let's first take a look at the gender distribution of the two diseases. This is where we see the most obvious difference in our daily clinical routine. Lipedema manifests itself almost exclusively in women. The cause of this remains unknown, despite increasing research in this area. Hormonal influences are considered to be the decisive factor. The frequent onset in phases of hormonal change, such as puberty, as well as the aggravation during pregnancy or even the late onset during menopause, speak in favor of this. If lipedema occurs in men, it is usually associated with other diseases (e.g., cirrhosis of the liver, hypogonadism) or is a side effect of hormonally active therapies (e.g., therapy of prostate carcinoma). Lymphedema, on the other hand, affects both men and women.

Cause
In contrast to lipedema, lymphedema has a tangible cause, namely either congenital (primary) or acquired (secondary) damage to the lymphatic transport system. This damage can, of course, vary greatly in its origin and severity. It should be noted that lymphedema (at least primary lymphedema) also occurs much more frequently in women than in men. Both diseases show a familial accumulation.

▶ Lipedema occurs almost exclusively in women, while lymphedema occurs in both men and women.

Affected Areas
A further difference can be seen in the external appearance of both clinical pictures. Although lipedema and lymphedema may look the same at first glance, since they share the symptom of swollen legs, ultimately a closer look at the affected areas usually reveals clear differences. While the swelling in lipedema always affects both legs or both arms, in lymphedema often only one leg or arm is affected by the increase in circumference. If in rare cases of lymphedema, swelling occurs on both sides, one side is usually more affected than the other. Feet and hands also show a clear difference in both clinical pictures. While the feet and hands are excluded from the swelling in lipedema, the backs of the feet and hands are usually clearly swollen in lymphedema (Fig. 2.13). This can be verified by a positive Stemmer's sign.

On the surface, lipedema is often accompanied by obesity, which places an increasing burden on those affected. Lymphedema, on the other hand, usually occurs independently of obesity, at least in the early stages.

Fig. 2.13 Swollen back of the hand in lymphedema

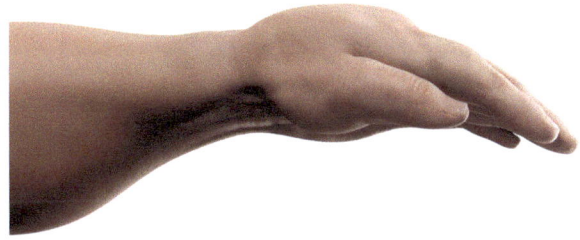

Palpation

During a closer examination in the course of our clinical examination, clear differences in the palpation findings of both diseases can also be observed. Lipedema appears mostly soft, often described as doughy or spongy. When the tissue is pressed in, no dent remains.

The tissue is similarly soft in early stages of lymphedema (stages 1 and 2). If we press the soft edema in lymphedema, a visible dent remains. In advanced lymphedema, where longer term edema deposits lead to increased collagen formation and thus to hardening of the tissue, pressing in is no longer possible.

Consequently, dents can only be depressed in "soft" lymphedema (early stages), but not in "soft" lipedema. In the late stages of lymphedema, the tissue is too hard to be depressed.

Skin Lesions

Further differences can be seen when looking at the skin of lipedema and lymphedema. The externally visible skin changes in lipedema are caused by the proliferation of fatty tissue under the skin without any actual structural change in the skin structure. In the early stages, the skin appears finely knotty, while a more coarseknotty appearance occurs in later stages.

In lymphedema, on the other hand, the protein-rich edema in advanced stages leads to structural changes in the skin and subcutis. Initially, there is a thickening of both the subcutis (i.e., the lower skin) and the cutis (skin), which is caused on the one hand by an increase in the subcutaneous fatty tissue and on the other hand by an increase in the connective tissue. Furthermore, trophic changes occur in the uppermost skin layer, the epidermis. The changes range from dry skin to hyperkeratosis, excessive growth of the uppermost skin layer, the already described hardening (pachyderma), often also called elephant skin, to the formation of areal skin tumors (papillomatosis), lymphatic vesicles, and ulcers.

Ultimately, the aforementioned skin changes in lymphedema, in combination with the impaired removal of lymphatic fluid, lead to damage to the natural skin barrier, which results in a significantly higher incidence of infections (e.g., erysipelas or cellulitis) in lymphedema than in lipedema.

Complaints

Let us now take a closer look at the complaints of both clinical pictures described by those affected. Here too, in addition to a few similarities, there are major differences between lipedema and lymphedema. It should be mentioned that the symptoms listed below represent only a cross section of the symptoms described by those affected. The occurrence is sometimes subject to strong individual variations.

Having said this, let's start with the similarities: First of all, what both diseases have in common is that the symptoms that occur significantly restrict the quality of life in everyday life and at work. For example, the increase in circumference can lead to restricted movement, which occurs in advanced stages of both diseases and is not infrequently so severe that the natural gait pattern appears to be significantly impeded.

In the case of lipedema, pain clearly dominates the symptoms of most of those affected. It should be clarified here that the currently valid staging does not take into account the painfulness of this disease. As a result, there is no direct correlation between stage and pain. This means that patients with stage I lipedema can subjectively experience significantly more pain than, for example, patients with stage III lipedema, but the same is also true the other way around—we have already discussed this topic several times in this context. Pain is described much less frequently in lymphedema and is more likely to occur in advanced stages or the case of complications such as erysipelas or cellulitis. The everyday limitations of lymphedema are mostly caused by the sensation of tension and heaviness.

Those affected by lipedema often report a strong sensitivity to touch, which is described rather rarely in lymphedema. The tendency to hematoma formation after minor trauma is also more likely to be attributed to lipedema than to lymphedema.

Apart from the obvious symptoms, sufferers of both conditions have to contend with severe restrictions in their everyday lives. For example, the usually one-sided swelling of lymphedema causes unexpected problems when buying clothes. Pants or tops usually have to be purchased several sizes too large to accommodate the one-sided swelling. Furthermore, the clothing often constricts the skin, which often causes problems due to the poor quality of the skin.

▶   In lipedema, the pain usually dominates the symptoms. These occur
      regardless of the respective stage. In lymphedema, these are usually
      only found in advanced stages.

Objectivity
Another striking difference is the objectifiability of both diseases. The basic diagnostic procedure, which is the same for both diseases and consists of anamnesis (questioning), inspection (examination) and palpation (palpation), allows the trained and experienced examiner to draw clear conclusions about the clinical picture. The distinction between lipedema and lymphedema seems to be relatively easy to make. But what about the distinction between lipohypertrophy and lipedema, whose only difference is the painfulness of the affected areas in lipedema? In this case, the examiner is solely dependent on the description of the affected person and can only make the diagnosis on the basis of his experience, examination, and statements of the affected person. Further diagnostics are simply not available when diagnosing lipedema. Unfortunately, the disease cannot be objectified in comparison to lymphedema, which makes it difficult for it to be recognized as a health insurance benefit. In the

case of lymphedema, on the other hand, we have numerous, so-called advanced diagnostic procedures at our disposal. In addition to morphological imaging procedures (MRI, CT, and ultrasound), these also include functional diagnostics (functional lymphoscintigraphy, indocyanine green lymphography) and various genetic tests.

▶   Lymphedema is objectifiable as a disease, lipedema is not.

Treatment
Although we will discuss therapy, especially that for lipedema, in detail in subsequent chapters, we will briefly discuss similarities and differences in both conditions.

Despite the commonality of CPE as a conservative therapeutic approach, it must again be made clear that lipedema and lymphedema are completely different clinical pictures. This is also the reason for the different therapy.

In lipedema, CPE only leads to an improvement of symptoms in some cases; a complete alleviation of symptoms by the combination of compression and lymphatic drainage is almost impossible. Particularly with regard to manual lymphatic drainage in lipedema, there is no proven effect. The only remaining therapeutic approach is liposuction, which, in our experience, greatly alleviates or completely eliminates the symptoms in almost all patients. It should be noted that even if the symptoms are completely reduced after surgical treatment of lipedema, it cannot be said that the disease has been cured. Also, a recurrence of the disease cannot be excluded by surgical therapy. The disease is therefore not curable.

In principle, CPD can achieve a significant improvement in the symptoms of lymphedema. In contrast to lipedema, manual lymphatic drainage represents a central point of therapy. It is also important to distinguish between congenital and acquired lymphedema. In addition to CPD, we now have numerous microsurgical procedures at our disposal, which can increasingly lead to a complete and, above all, permanent reduction in symptoms and even cure.

The differences between lipedema and lymphedema are shown in Fig. 2.14.

We do not want to leave unmentioned that there are also mixed pictures of these diseases among themselves or with other diseases. Lipo-lymphoedema and phlebo-lymphoedema should be mentioned in particular. We have already discussed obesity.

As the name suggests, lipolymphedema is a mixed form of lipedema and lymphedema. In some patients, lymphedema also develops during the course of lipedema (Fig. 2.15). In addition to the typical symptoms of lipedema, there are also symptoms of lymphedema that are not usually found in lipedema. An example of this is the swollen backs of the feet or hands or edema on the lower legs that can be pushed away. In contrast to pure lymphedema, the edema in lipo-lymphedema is usually symmetrical.

In Fig. 2.16 marked lipo-lymphoedema after massive weight loss is shown.

Phlebo-lymphedema is a combination of venous disease and lymphedema. It is caused by chronic venous insufficiency, a venous outflow obstruction that can be caused, for example, by varicose veins, phlebothrombosis, or arteriovenous malformations. This damage to the veins can result in the blood not returning properly from the periphery of the body back to the heart. The blood backs up, so to speak, and presses fluid out of the veins into the surrounding tissue.

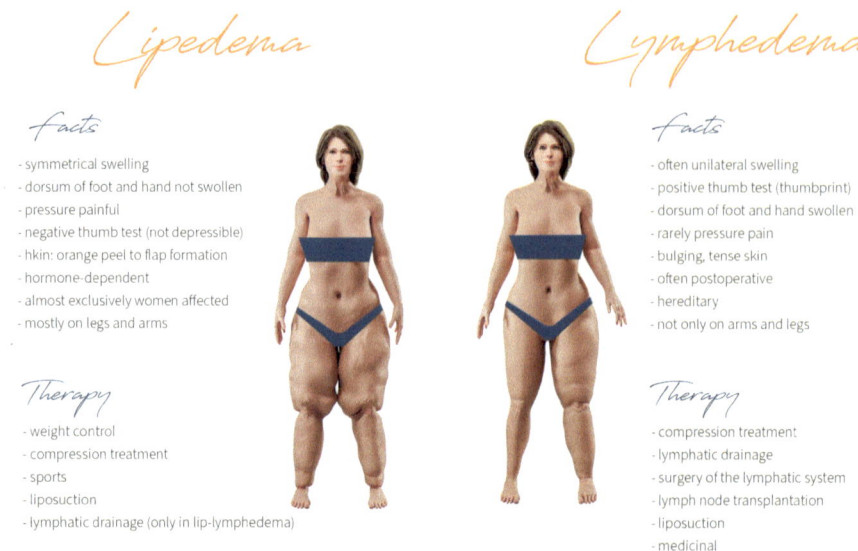

Lipedema

facts

- symmetrical swelling
- dorsum of foot and hand not swollen
- pressure painful
- negative thumb test (not depressible)
- hkin: orange peel to flap formation
- hormone-dependent
- almost exclusively women affected
- mostly on legs and arms

Therapy

- weight control
- compression treatment
- sports
- liposuction
- lymphatic drainage (only in lip-lymphedema)

Lymphedema

facts

- often unilateral swelling
- positive thumb test (thumbprint)
- dorsum of foot and hand swollen
- rarely pressure pain
- bulging, tense skin
- often postoperative
- hereditary
- not only on arms and legs

Therapy

- compression treatment
- lymphatic drainage
- surgery of the lymphatic system
- lymph node transplantation
- liposuction
- medicinal

Fig. 2.14 Differences between lipedema and lymphedema

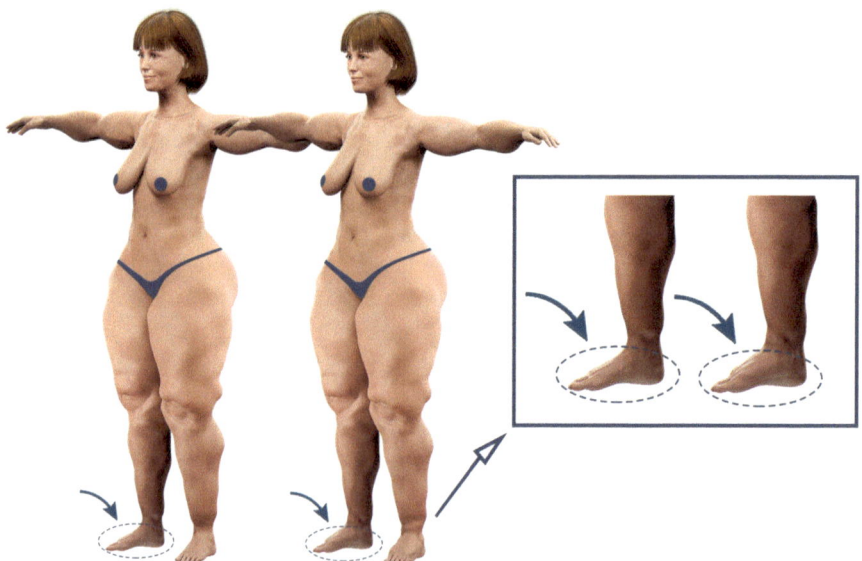

Fig. 2.15 Dorsal edema of the foot in lymphedema

As a consequence, increased tissue fluid is produced here as well, which—similar to lipo-lymphoedema—leads to an overload of the lymphatic vascular system. In phlebo-lymphoedema, too, early treatment of the underlying disease is indispensable. Manual lymphatic drainage and compression therapy are prescribed as supportive measures.

Fig. 2.16 Lipo-
lymphedema after massive
weight loss

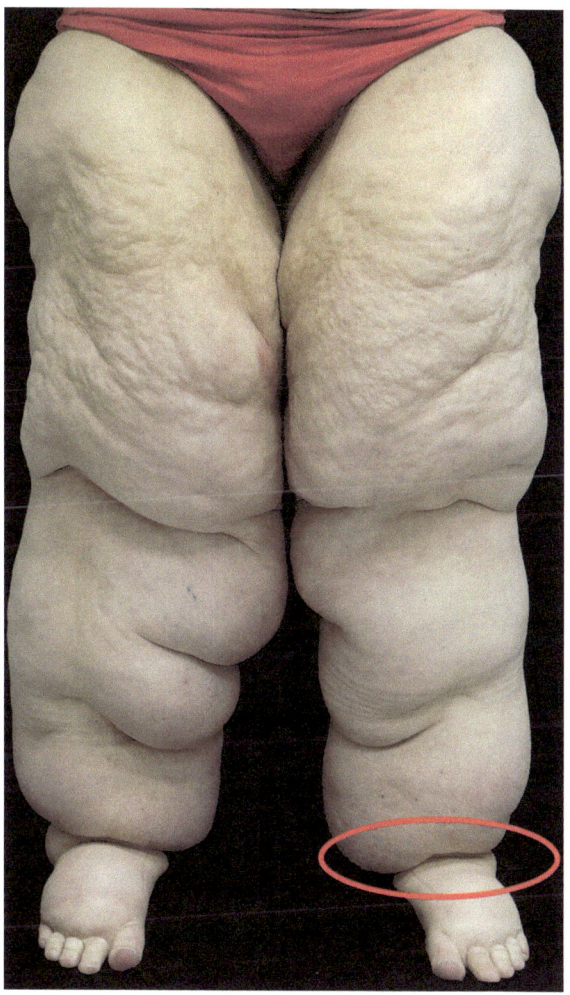

There is another very impressive observation from our daily surgical routine when we compare lipedema and lymphedema. When we take a patient with lymphedema to the operating room and make a skin incision, tissue water (edema) escapes from the wound immediately after penetration of the skin with the scalpel. Occasionally, this edema discharge can be observed through the skin suture into the dressing for several days after the operation. The situation is completely different in lipedema. Although a small incision must be made through the skin at the beginning of every liposuction procedure, we have never seen even a drop of tissue water leak out in lipedema in the past 15 years.

Basic differences and similarities between lipedema and lymphedema are summarized here.

1. Lipedema and lymphedema are two entirely different conditions, both of which cause swollen legs.

2. Lipedema occurs almost exclusively in women, while lymphedema occurs in both men and women.
3. Lipedema always shows a symmetrical swelling. Lymphedema often shows asymmetric swelling of an arm or leg.
4. In lymphedema, the backs of the hands and/or feet are also affected by swelling, but not lipedema.
5. Stemmer's sign is negative in lipedema but positive in lymphedema.
6. The swelling in lipedema feels soft, in advanced lymphedema, it is hard and bulging.
7. In lipedema, the pain usually dominates the symptoms. It occurs regardless of the respective stage. In lymphedema, pain is usually observed only in advanced stages.
8. Common complications of advanced lymphedema are erysipelas (erysipelas) and cellulitis. These do not usually occur in lipedema.
9. A tendency to hematoma formation is observed in lipedema, even after minor trauma, but not in lymphedema.
10. Lymphedema is caused by a disorder of the lymphatic transport system. The cause of the development of lipedema is not clear to date.
11. Obesity can lead to the development of lymphedema. In lipedema, it can have a negative effect on progression and also be associated with it.
12. Lymphedema can usually be diagnosed causally with diagnostic imaging procedures. There is no apparative examination that is conclusive for lipedema.
13. Both diseases may or may not progress. Whether in what time frame or to what extent the diseases progress cannot be predicted for both lipedema and lymphedema.
14. Manual lymphatic drainage is a core element of lymphedema therapy. In lipedema, it usually has no lasting effect.
15. In both diseases, it is important to treat not only the physical effects but also the psychological stress.

References

Campisi CC, Villa G et al (2019) Rationale for the study of the deep subfascial lymphatic vessels during lymphoscintigraphy for the diagnosis of peripheral lymphedema. Clin Nucl Med 44:91–98
Campisi C, Ryan M, Campisi CS, Boccardo F, Campisi CC (2018) Lymphatic Venous Anastomosis Applied in the Surgical Management of Peripheral Lymphedema: from Prophylaxis to Advanced Disease. In H-C Chen, P Ciudad, S-H Chen, YB Tang. Lymphedema Surgical Approaches and Specific Topics (Chapter 6, pp. 55–70). Elsevier. 2nd edition
Campisi C, Marlys W et al (2020) Matching Primary with Secondary Lymphedemas across Lymphatic Surgery in Genoa Italy from 1973 until time of Covid 19. Italian Journal of Vascular and Endovascular Surgery, Minerva Medica 2021(March);28(1):25–41.
Villa G, Campisi CC, Campisi C et al (2019) Procedural recommendations for lymphoscintigraphy in the diagnosis of peripheral lymphedema: the Genoa Protocol. Nuclear Medicine and Molecular Imaging 53:47–56

Treatment of Lipedema

Zaher Jandali, Benedikt Merwart, Ralf Weise,
Angel Pecorelli Capozzi, and Lucian Jiga

3.1   Introduction

In our opinion, lipedema has serious consequences for those affected. In addition to the pain, which is often responsible for a high level of suffering, mobility and overall resilience are often significantly limited. The heavy weight-bearing associated with lipedema can lead to painful wear and tear in the hip and knee joints at an early stage. Those affected withdraw, feel misunderstood, marginalized, or even discriminated against. These social and psychosocial components have a major impact. We have an obligation not only to treat the pain but also to reintegrate those affected into social life. We must help to make possible a life free of psychological pressure.

It is important that all doctors take the complaints of those affected very seriously and do not simply continue the "fat leg principle" as before. It is not enough to tell sufferers that weight loss is the right thing to do and that they should just eat less. If it were that simple, sufferers would have already done it. Sufferers need to feel taken seriously and well cared for.

We see a colorful landscape of different players with different training, orientation, and interest in the treatment of lipedema. We see that the market is highly competitive, with oral and maxillofacial surgeons, orthopedic surgeons, gynecologists, vascular surgeons, and dermatologists presenting themselves as experts in lipedema. This is not at all objectionable, as everyone can contribute something to

Z. Jandali (✉) · B. Merwart · L. Jiga
Department of Plastic, Aesthetic, Reconstructive and Hand Surgery, Evangelical Hospital
Oldenburg, Oldenburg, Niedersachsen, Germany
e-mail: dr@jandali.de

R. Weise
Klinik für Allgemein- und Visceralchirurgie, St. Marienhospital Friesoythe gemeinnützige
GmbH, Friesoythe, Germany

A. P. Capozzi
PLATINUM MEDICAL CENTER, SLP, Carrer Sant Elíes, entresuelo 115, Barcelona, Spain

© Springer Nature Switzerland AG 2022
Z. Jandali et al. (eds.), *Lipedema*, https://doi.org/10.1007/978-3-030-86717-1_3

the cure and research from their area of expertise. However, what makes one wonder greatly is that few are concerned with conservative treatment and instead turn to surgical liposuction.

Quite aggressive advertising is used for this. To outdo each other, there is a real power struggle with tempting offers containing false statements. It can almost be described as "normal" when doctors hire professional bloggers to specifically advertise for them. When we read on the tempting web portals: "Lipedema is curable," "We cure lipedema," or "We suck off all the fatty tissue, with us no fat remains," we wonder what is going wrong. On the point, some drive it then, which want to generate a patient influx with the stoking of fears: "If you do not let yourselves be sucked off, then it becomes always worse." This statement is then underlined by the publication of rare lipedema pictures, which are to be seen as the final stage and the evil to be expected. We are particularly uncomfortable with bloggers and hired laymen working under the guise of nonprofit.

We will tell you how to find a good, reputable, and practically trained doctor in Chap. 5. Even we, the authors of the book, are not the measure of all things, but we will try to give you an honest picture of the nevertheless opaque situation and the pronounced conflict of interests of the individual players. Don't fall for it. "We will cure your lipedema," sounds good, but it is not true.

We even go a small step further. In Germany, for example, even politicians have put on the shoe of wanting to take care of lipedema sufferers—an approach that is very much to be welcomed. However, politics has placed itself in a nest of nettles. Instead of promoting and supporting research, liposuction in certain stages of lipedema is now covered by health insurance in Germany. From our point of view, this is a gross and negligent injustice for all those who do not fall into the stages. In addition, the stage-dependent surgical indication, based on a purely descriptive classification of stages, can hardly be surpassed in nonsense and cannot be verified by any objective means. Here, too, politicians, driven by bloggers and clueless laymen, only want to put themselves in the center of events and do not want to take care of the affected persons in a sustainable way.

We stand for evidence in medicine, and in lipedema, there is simply almost none. This also applies to all our statements, which are based on experience and very few good studies. Those who work at the grassroots level are the real heroes in our view. These include the doctors in research who are working on this issue with few financial resources, the self-help groups with their tireless efforts to support those affected, and the many honest doctors who do not have a microphone in front of their mouths all day to communicate. The truth of it all is, as always, somewhere in between.

When we think about what good treatment of patients with lipedema looks like, we have to take a holistic view of the patient and the options available to us. In addition to the therapy of the pain, which should be in the foreground, any existing secondary diseases must also be treated. This may include obesity or mental illnesses such as depression.

Let's talk about the treatment options. The basic prerequisite for us as treatment providers is that the desire for treatment comes from you personally. Only then will you also have the necessary motivation and discipline to experience long-term success.

Just a few months ago, a mother and her daughter came to see me. Right from the start, the mother had the floor and began by saying that she had seen a report on television and had known right away that she herself and also her daughter would suffer from lipedema. She had always wondered why she looked the way she did and wanted to spare her young daughter these thoughts. When asked how her daughter saw it, she said that she had noticed for a long time that her proportions were not quite right either, but that it had never bothered her. Neither she nor her mother had any pain. There is no lipedema, but a simple lipohypertrophy. The young daughter does not wish to undergo treatment. It, therefore, makes no sense to treat the daughter. It would make more sense to possibly treat the mother, but then for aesthetic reasons and not on the basis of lipedema.

The path of any treatment is complex, whether conservative or surgical. In most cases, existing pain can be treated well by whatever method. Certainly, there are also rare therapy-refractory courses (courses that do not respond to therapy), but ultimately our experience shows that almost all sufferers can be relieved of their pain. Perhaps not always with the measures that the affected person would like, but there are possibilities. The outside can also always be positively influenced. It just depends on what goals the sufferers have, how realistic they are, and what they are willing to put in to achieve the goals. A statement like "I was told that no one can help me" is certainly only understandable in the case of severe secondary illnesses or other special reasons. Other questions include medical necessity and who will pay the costs.

Let's take another look at the group of lipedema sufferers (Fig. 3.1). Since more than 50% of lipedema sufferers also suffer from morbid obesity, long-term treatment of obesity is often a crucial component in the treatment of lipedema. The primary goal is to prevent further weight gain or, in the best case, to bring about weight reduction, depending on the initial weight.

Different treatment aspects can be considered for the treatment of lipedema. These are in detail:

1. Conservative treatment.
   a. Weight stabilization (nutritional therapy and lifestyle adjustment).
   b. Compression treatment.
   c. Manual lymphatic drainage (only if edema is present).
   d. Apparative lymphatic drainage (only if edema is present).
   e. Exercise therapy.
2. Complex surgical treatment.
   a. Weight stabilization (conservative or surgical).
   b. Liposuction for lipedema treatment.
   c. Lifting operations according to need and medical necessity.

Since we find weight stabilization in all treatment concepts, we will first discuss it. If you have an extreme fat distribution disorder and are of normal weight or only slightly to moderately overweight, you can skip Sect. 3.2.

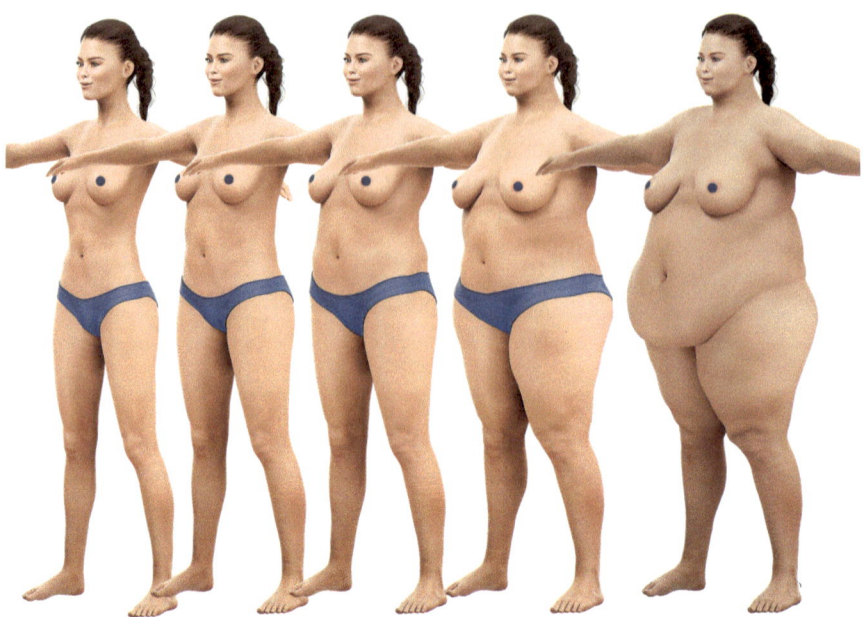

Fig. 3.1 Normal to severely overweight body shapes (without fat distribution disorder)

3.2 Measures for Weight Stabilization

In weight stabilization measures, we distinguish conservative from surgical measures. Let's start with the general and conservative measures.

3.2.1 Conservative Measures

In this context, it seems important to us to point out that the change of diet should be clearly distinguished from a diet. Perhaps you have already been on many unsuccessful diets. If you still have doubts in this regard, let us tell you: Diets are NOT the right way! But why? Often the problem lies in the way we lose weight. Low-calorie diets often do not lead to weight loss, but weight gain in the aftermath. What is the mechanism? With diets where we only eat 1000–1200 kcal per day, the pounds may well fall off at the beginning of such a diet, but as soon as the desired weight is reached (or not), the well-known yo-yo effect occurs.

The reason for this is that we initially lose mainly muscle mass. Lack of muscle mass leads to a reduction in basal metabolic rate. With the same food intake as before the diet, there is a continuous weight gain due to the now lower muscle mass. There is further scientific evidence as to why weight increases after dieting. The blood leptin level after a low kilojoule diet decreases. The low leptin level causes an increase in appetite. At the same time, metabolism slows down. The increase in appetite and slowing of metabolism can support this yo-yo effect.

▶ We do not recommend dieting.

The repeated weight gain after diets has also given rise to the popular opinion that lipedema is diet-resistant. This cannot be generalized in this way. In general, the lower the obesity and the greater the disproportion, the smaller the effect of weight loss on the areas affected by lipedema. In normal-weight lipedema sufferers, weight loss will accordingly bring only a small change, sometimes only visible at a second glance.

▶ We do not agree with the common opinion that areas affected by lipedema cannot be influenced by weight loss.

The explanation for this probably lies in the altered hormonal responsiveness and signal processing of the fat cells. The diseased adipose tissue appears to be more resistant to weight loss than the adipose tissue in other regions. It decreases disproportionately to the residual adipose tissue during weight loss. But again, it's different for overweight or severely obese people. Here, a prolonged and permanent weight loss is certainly accompanied by an overall decrease of the excess adipose tissue, including the areas of disproportion and the painful areas of lipedema. In many cases, weight loss is also accompanied by a significant improvement in pain symptoms, sometimes more, sometimes less pronounced. One of the most common statements made by sufferers is: "When I lose weight, it's everywhere but on my legs and arms. "We do not agree with this, as we must again take into account the different starting conditions.

▶ Massive weight loss in sufferers with a BMI >40 kg/m2 is often accompanied by relief of the pain associated with lipedema.

Let's now ask the loaded question: If a large percentage of lipedema sufferers also suffer from obesity, how well can they lose weight on their own? The answer is: very poorly! About 95% of all self-directed diet attempts in sufferers with a BMI >40 kg/m^2 fail. That's a statement you have to come to terms with first. So if you have lipedema and a BMI >40 kg/m^2, it is very likely that you will not be able to lose weight on your own. You need professional help to treat your obesity.

Whenever we feel that there is significant obesity, we recommend treating it as a first step. Depending on the degree of obesity, there are different approaches to treat it.

This book is not a nutritional guide, but lipedema is associated with overweight or obesity in the majority of patients. Therefore, we cannot hide the issue therapeutically and have to deal with it. This is not about dieting, but about changing lifestyle habits and eating behavior. We will be brief at this point, as there are separate books and guidebooks for this.

The causes of obesity are complex and not easy to break down. In the first step, it is important to visualize your ideal "I" internally. What characteristics should your ideal "I" have? This is about behaviors, attitudes (e.g., about food and exercise), and where you see your body. How is the ideal "me" different from your current, present "me"? What are the lifestyle habits you would like to have?

After a little self-reflection, you will find your answer. You should recognize and implement the challenges that this poses to you. In the next step, it is important to summarize the experiences you have made so far. Regardless of your success, it is the journey that counts. Don't value your results so far as failures, but as steps that bring you closer to your goal. Methods that don't work for you bring you closer to those that do.

What measures do we recommend when we talk about changing eating habits? There are thousands of different ways. But this much from our side: we do not recommend a dietary change that should work purely by reducing the number of calories. To be successful, an adjustment must be made in four key areas of life: Nutrition, fitness, lifestyle, and psychology (Table 3.1).

The need for additional psychological co-treatment should be discussed with each patient and initiated if necessary.

Did you know that there are many concepts that attribute incredible weight loss potential to the vital substance-rich fresh diet? It is even possible for someone suffering from obesity to lose weight on a hypercaloric diet, as long as the diet contains enough vital substances to make this reduction.

Table 3.1 Measures per key area for a lasting change in diet

Area	Measure
Nutrition	Refrain from fats as far as possible
	Reduce carbohydrates/sugar to the maximum (avoid sweets, soft drinks, dough products such as bread or spaghetti)
	Conduct your dietary changes in a way that you don't think of them as diets, but as long-term dietary changes
	Exercise at least 20 min daily with an increase to 30 min
	To do this, find a sport that you enjoy (alternate muscle building/cardio workouts)
Fitness	Increase daily activity
	Walk paths
Lifestyle	Avoid elevators
	Your work must leave you room for cooking, sports, and balance
	Rethink your sleep patterns
	Surround yourself with healthy living people
	If the people around you oppose you, hinder you, or slow you down, think about these relationships
	Analyze imbalances related to work, family, relationship, and finances
	Think positive
Psychology	Reduce stress to avoid relapse
	Love yourself and others
	Have grace toward yourself. Don't give up right away if you don't reach the goal once. Nobody is perfect
	Write in a diary. This helps to reflect
	Think long term. Short-term goals do not lead to the desired result

3.2.2 Surgical Measures for Weight Stabilization

Ralf Weise

Because conservative measures have a high failure rate for weight loss, surgical measures for weight stabilization have been at the forefront for some time. Patients with morbid obesity are high-risk patients. The demanding treatment requires close cooperation of many disciplines, which can only be guaranteed at specialized centers.

Several months usually pass from the first contact to the implementation of an operative procedure, during which numerous examinations and treatments as well as organizational measures take place. For the planning and implementation of such a demanding concept, structured treatment paths as well as an institution that takes over the management of the patients and the organization have proven their worth. Such an institution for the treatment of patients with obesity-related diseases is called an obesity center.

Obesity centers at large urban hospitals or university hospitals usually have all the necessary specialist groups under one roof. In contrast, obesity centers in smaller hospitals, some of which are located in rural areas, often have to rely on external cooperation partners. In these centers with a large catchment area, follow-up care can also be organized close to home at external locations. Both concepts are possible and can demonstrate comparably good long-term results.

Numerous studies and follow-up observations over the past decades have shown that a lifelong change in lifestyle only succeeds in absolutely exceptional cases without professional help. However, even with professional support, weight regain often occurs after treatment.

When the nonsurgical approaches to the treatment of morbid obesity remain unsuccessful and have been exhausted, it is time to consider so-called metabolic interventions to support the therapy. As the name suggests, these are surgeries that serve to treat the secondary diseases of obesity, metabolic disorders. The additional reduction of body weight is a means to an end.

Based on numerous study results, there is worldwide agreement among experts on when surgery should be offered. The current German guidelines are also based on this scheme.

Surgical therapy for obesity is used when all nonsurgical treatment options have failed to achieve the treatment goal and one of the following constellations is present:

1. BMI between 30 and 35 kg/m^2 in patients with particular severity of concomitant and secondary diseases of obesity,
2. BMI between 35 and 40 kg/m^2 with secondary diseases (e.g., diabetes mellitus, hypertension),
3. BMI of 40 kg/m^2 or higher.

From a BMI of 50 kg/m^2, there is an absolute reason to include a surgical procedure in the treatment plan.

Before undergoing metabolic surgery, every patient should participate in a preparation program. There is a whole range of different surgical procedures for the treatment of obesity, i.e. metabolic interventions, which are used worldwide. Many of these procedures are performed only sporadically in some centers. Their long-term benefit is often not sufficiently proven. Therefore, only the currently established procedures will be presented here. In advance, you will see the normal anatomy shown in Fig. 3.2.

All interventions are based on two effects, which are used either alone or in combination:

– Reduction of the volume of ingested food by reducing the size of the stomach.
– Reduction of absorption of food components in the small intestine due to bypassing of the small intestine.

Which surgical procedure is the right one must be decided on an individual basis. The choice of surgical procedure depends, among other things, on the patient's eating habits, underlying diseases of the gastrointestinal tract, and occupational and lifestyle habits.

Adjustable Gastric Band

A plastic band is placed around the upper part of the stomach (Fig. 3.3). This band is connected via a tube to a can which is positioned under the skin. By puncturing this can with a special needle, the size of the band can be adjusted. Thus, the patient's personal setting, his "green zone," must be found in several sessions.

The number of gastric band implantations has declined sharply in Europe in recent years, while this procedure was first approved in the United States in 2010 and initially experienced a real boom there.

Even though this is a quick, low-risk surgical procedure, many complications, most of them minor, often occur as the procedure progresses. These range from slipping of the band to infections and ingrowth of the band into the stomach. In

Fig. 3.2 The normal anatomy of the gastrointestinal tract

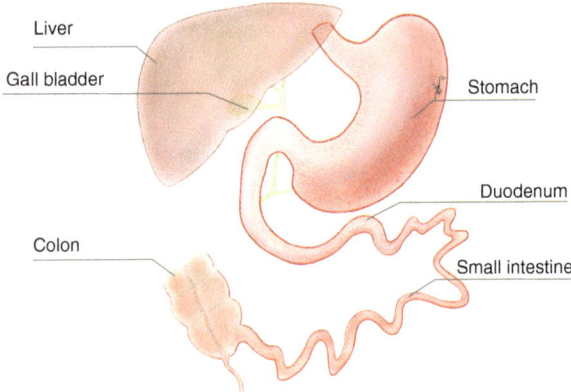

Fig. 3.3 Adjustable gastric band with port system

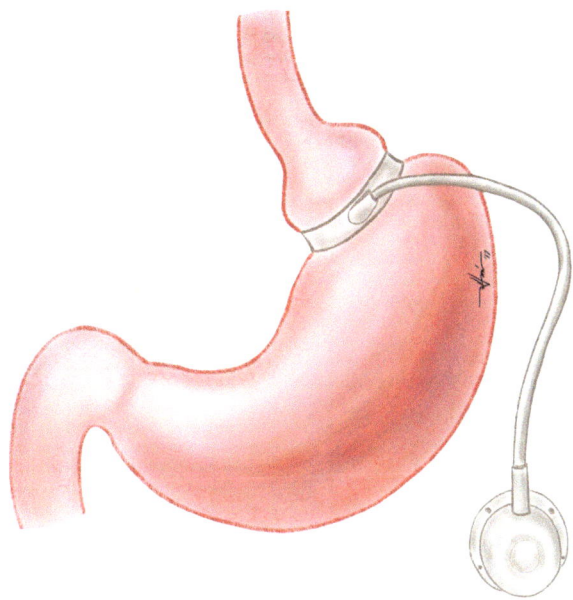

addition, the cooperation of the patient and regular follow-up care are particularly important with this procedure in order to achieve long-lasting good results.

Many gastric bands must therefore be removed again in the course of life. Since the problem of obesity then persists, another procedure usually has to be performed.

Gastric Tube (Sleeve Resection)

The entire length of the stomach is closed and cut, leaving only a narrow tube (Fig. 3.4). In contrast to other metabolic procedures, a large part (approx. 2/3) of the stomach must be removed. During the procedure, a relatively wide gastric tube is placed in the stomach so that the gastric tube does not become too narrow.

Gastric sleeve formation has been increasingly used to treat morbid obesity for about 15 years. In 2017, over 60% of metabolic procedures in Germany were sleeve resections. Originally, gastric sleeve was a precursor to performing a more complex procedure. However, it has become increasingly established as a treatment procedure in its own right in recent years.

This procedure is only suitable to a limited extent for patients with heartburn (a so-called reflux disease). Recent studies on this topic are currently causing a critical rethinking of this surgical technique.

Gastric Bypass

The stomach is separated in the upper region (Fig. 3.5), leaving only a small residual stomach for the passage of food. For the onward passage of the food, the small intestine is cut at a certain point and connected to the small stomach. The previously severed small intestine, which is attached to the large stomach remnant, is reconnected to the small intestine at a lower point.

Fig. 3.4 Sleeve resection

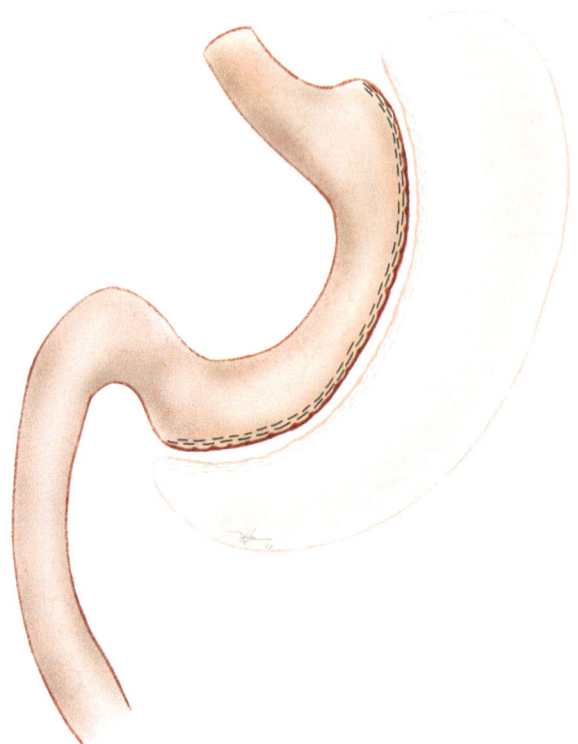

Fig. 3.5 Gastric bypass

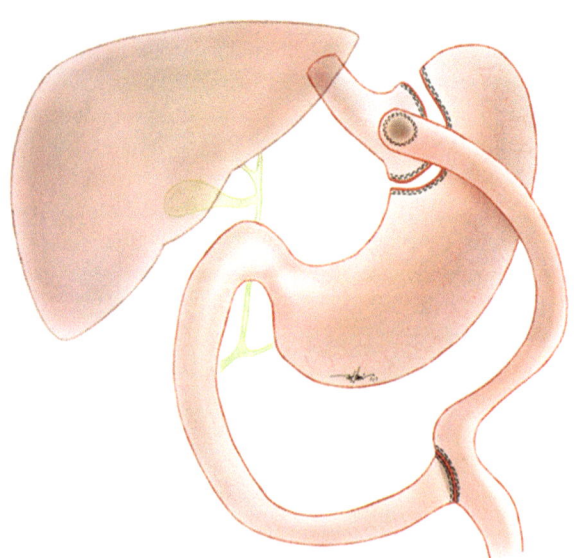

As a rule, this procedure achieves a weight reduction of 50–70% of excess weight. It combines stomach reduction with small intestine bypass.

The first described insertion of a gastric bypass for the treatment of morbid obesity took place in 1966 by MD Mason in the United States. Since then, this procedure has become established, initially in North America and in recent years also in many other countries.

The gastric bypass procedure is the best compromise for many patients because of the low risk of surgery and a high quality of life, as well as its excellent impact on secondary diseases. Under the regular intake of vitamins and trace elements, there is only a small risk of developing malnutrition.

Mini Bypass (Omega Loop)

The stomach is severed in the middle region, leaving only a relatively small residual stomach for the passage of food (Fig. 3.6). To pass the food on, a loop of small intestine is connected to the side of the small stomach at a specific point.

It combines a stomach reduction with a bypass of the small intestine. Some substances in food, especially fats and carbohydrates, are no longer absorbed by the intestine to the same extent as before the operation.

The Omega Loop is a relatively new procedure and has been used for several years with increasing numbers of operations. Even though it is now an established procedure, its position in the 2020 round of metabolic interventions has not yet been defined with certainty.

Duodenal Switch

After creation of a tubular stomach (sleeve), the duodenum is cut behind the stomach outlet. For the unobstructed passage of food, a connection is made between the

Fig. 3.6 Omega loop

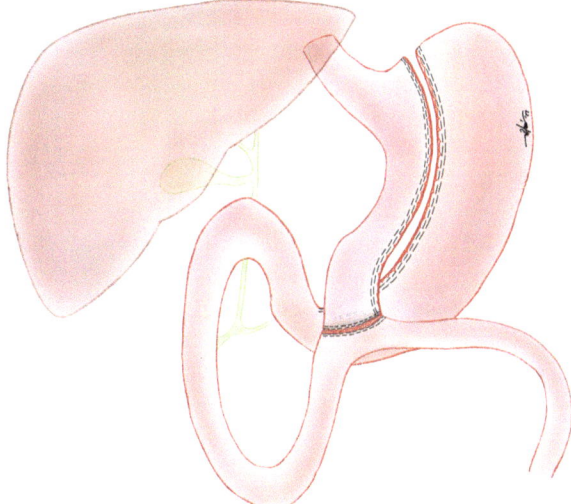

Fig. 3.7 Duodenal switch

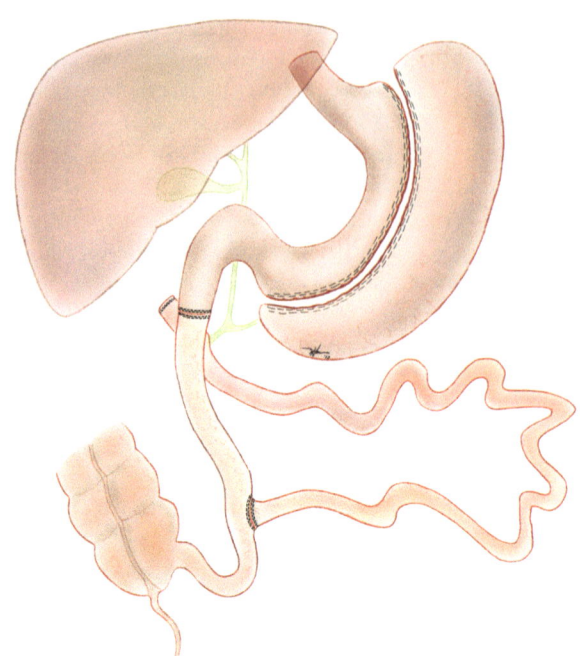

stomach and small intestine after the small intestine has been cut. The remaining loose end of the small intestine, which carries crucial digestive juices, is connected to the colon relatively close to the point where the small intestine joins the colon (Fig. 3.7).

As a rule, this procedure achieves a weight reduction of more than 70% of excess weight. In contrast to gastric bypass, the gastric pylorus is preserved, which reduces the risk of food falling out. It is occasionally performed as a second surgical treatment step after sleeve resection.

With a reduction of over 70% in excess weight and excellent control of concomitant diseases, patients with a duodenal switch have the best long-term outcomes.

SADI-S

The duodenal switch procedure is surgically demanding with a significantly increased complication rate. An alternative procedure has therefore been developed in which a gastric tube is also formed. In contrast to the duodenal switch, a loop of small intestine is connected laterally to the duodenum beyond the gastric outlet to pass the food (Fig. 3.8). The operation times and the risk of complications are thus significantly lower than with the duodenal switch.

The relatively radical small bowel bypasses of the last two procedures lead more frequently than the other procedures to malnutrition and occasionally to foul-smelling fatty stools. They are therefore considered reserve procedures for particularly severe courses of disease.

Fig. 3.8 SADI-S

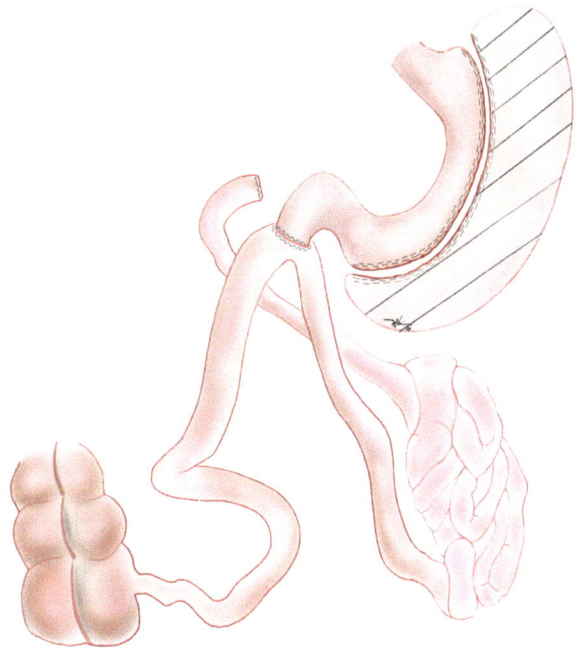

3.3   Complex Physical Therapy

Let's talk about the complex-physical therapy of lipedema. It consists of the following components:

- Compression treatment.
- Manual lymphatic drainage (only if edema is present).
- Apparative lymphatic drainage (only if edema is present).
- Exercise Therapy.
- Rehabilitation treatment.

Certainly, complex-physical therapy is an important component of treatment, and we have often observed an improvement through a change in lifestyle with appropriate dietary changes and exercise in combination with complex-physical therapy, but rather only discretely pronounced. In addition, we have not yet seen lipedema regress via physical treatment.

Compression Treatment
Normally, compression treatment is given to reduce edema, i.e. typically in lymphedema and lipo-lymphedema. By reducing the edema, there is a decrease in symptoms. In lipedema, the situation is different, since in the majority of cases there is no edema. Consequently, the edema is not the reason for the compression treatment. There is evidence for a reduced pain stimulus transmission triggered by the

compression treatment and thus pain reduction. In addition, the compression garment gives a feeling of stability.

The question that often arises is: flat knitted or circular knitted compression stockings? Circular or flat knitted refers to the manufacturing process. Circular knitted stockings are made seamless and spiral. They are more elastic and give more than flat knitted ones. Flat knitted stockings are made of more robust material and with a seam. Flat knitted stockings can exert pressure over a wider area, are more individually adjustable, and are also suitable for difficult conditions.

Venous disorders are usually treated with round-knitted compression stockings. In contrast, patients with edema are more likely to receive flat-knit compression stockings. Flat-knit compression stockings have also proven effective for lipedema. Compression stockings are available in different compression classes. We distinguish between compression classes 1–4, with compression class 1 being the lightest and 4 the strongest (Table 3.2).

In compression garments, we distinguish between custom-made and prefabricated compression garments. In addition, different forms of compression garments are available. Classic for lipedema are stockings in a long form and—much rarer—in a short form (Figs. 3.9 and Fig. 3.10).

However, most often we see compression tights. From our experience, we have the best feedback from tights (including the hips), as they fit quite stably and provide good comfort. The form of compression used depends on the areas and how pronounced the lipedema is.

A compression garment for lipedema is available through a prescription from a panel physician, including a change of care. All those who do not suffer from clinical edema and start compression treatment will notice a reduction in circumference when wearing compression garments. In combination with the loss of inherent elasticity of the compression pants, a replacement fitting is necessary after approximately 6 months—possibly earlier for the first fitting.

Due to the individual characteristics, we recommend custom-made flat-knitted compression stockings class II in the form of pantyhose. Most medical supply stores will measure you individually for this. Sleeves or boleros (jackets) are available for the arms. Here we rather recommend the use of boleros.

▶   For lipedema, we recommend a supply of flat-knitted compression stockings class II.

Table 3.2 Compression stocking classes

Compression class	Strength	Compression in kPA	Compression in mmHG
I	Easy	2.4–2.8	18–21
II	Medium	3.1–4.3	23–32
III	Powerful	4.5–6.1	34–46
IV	Very strong	>6.5	>49

Fig. 3.9 Compression stockings short (lower leg stockings)

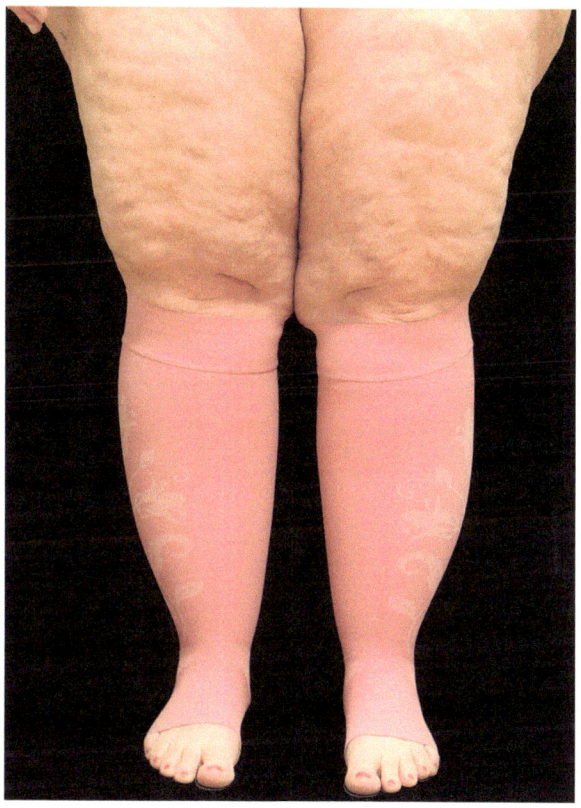

Manual Lymphatic Drainage

If there is no edema, no drainage of this edema can be responsible for pain relief. However, many state that lymphatic drainage relieves pain and does good. So what is the positive effect of lymphatic drainage? The positive effect of lymphatic drainage probably lies more in the attention experienced through therapy. The closeness to the therapist, the recognition of the disease, and accompanying processing. The therapist is there for you, listens and is a constant contact person for your illness. Those affected can often switch off and "shut down" in the process.

▷   Even if lymphatic drainage has positive effects, they are not due to the treatment of the disease.

Apparative Lymphatic Drainage

Apparatus lymphatic drainage, also known as apparatus intermittent compression (AIK) or intermittent pneumatic compression (IPC), is often colloquially referred to as "lymphomat" and is not indicated for classic lipedema. Apparative lymphatic drainage is regularly used in decongestive therapy for lymphatic or venous diseases. If lipo-lymphedema exists, lymphatic drainage by means of an apparatus makes sense.

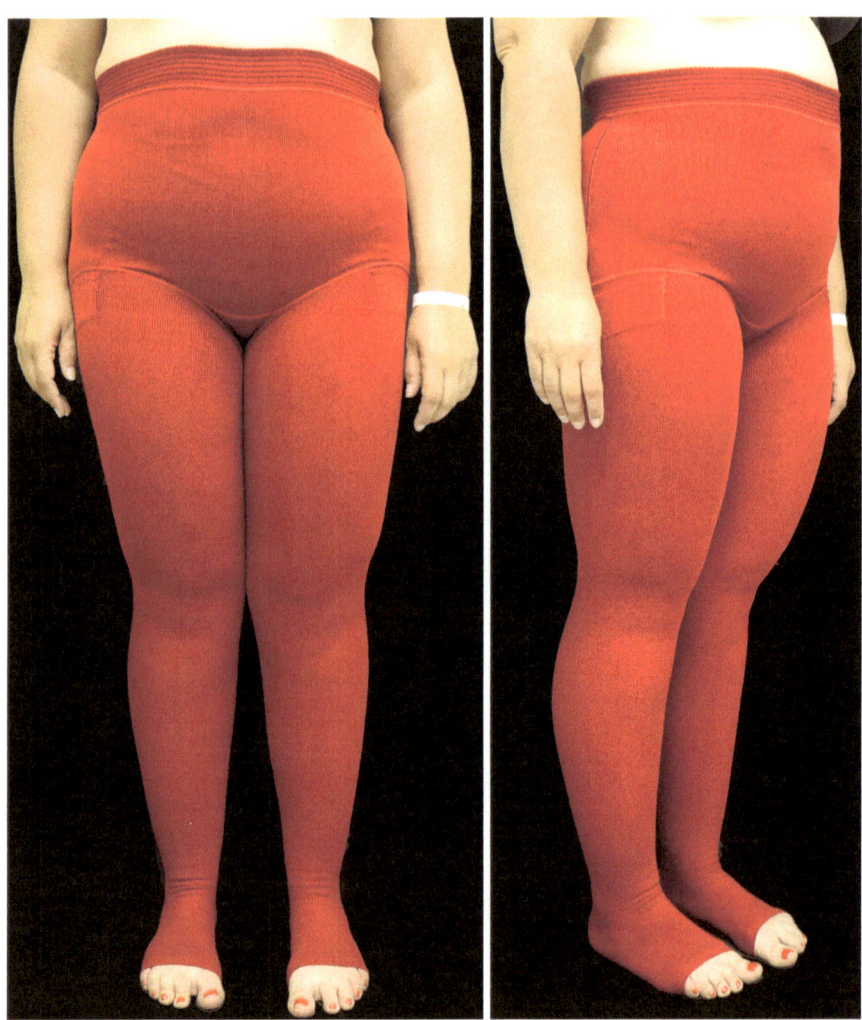

Fig. 3.10 Compression tights long

This is how apparative lymphatic drainage works: A double-walled cuff consisting of several air chambers are applied to the legs or arms and connected to a programmed compressor. The compressor regulates the air supply and discharge as well as air pressure in the cuff. The device generates pressure up to 200 mmHg. The pumping cycles are programmed to cause decongestion. The cuff pumps up first away from the body and then the overlapping air chambers. The chambers remain filled until the last chamber reaches the set pressure. Then simultaneous deflation occurs and a new cycle begins.

The devices are available in practices and for home use. A prescription is issued by the doctor. The medical supply store then checks whether the costs are covered by the health insurance company and finally provides the device. This method also uses external pressure to support the veins and lymphatic vessels.

▶ Apparative decongestive therapy is not a basic therapy for lipedema and is reserved for diseases with an edema component.

Exercise Therapy
As an essential component, we would like to mention exercise therapy. By this we mean an increase in activity and muscle building. Initially, exercise in and around water, e.g. aqua walking and aqua gymnastics, is certainly advisable due to the reduction of the patient's own weight in the water and simultaneous water resistance. Water-based exercise therapy is gentle on the joints and sustainable. It is also important here that not only fitness but also musculature is built up.

There are experts and further literature for movement therapy to which we would like to refer at this point. A highly recommended program for exercise and fitness in general is, for example, the so-called Sei-stolz-auf-dich concept (www.seistolza-ufdich.de).

Rehabilitation Treatment
Initial treatment with a holistic approach often takes place during inpatient rehabilitation treatment (cure). Here, depending on the concept, the psyche and body are strengthened. Furthermore, nutritional counseling and decongestion therapy are often provided. Certainly, rehab is more indicated for those affected with edema than for those without, since the initial edema therapy requires constant and daily treatment.

3.4   Complex Surgical Treatment

In the past, surgical therapy for lipedema was always in the background and was the last therapeutic option, even for us surgeons. I still remember my first day of plastic surgery training. One of my first patients in the consultation was actually a lipedema patient. At that time, metabolic surgery was still in its infancy, and we often performed so-called megaliposuctions in which many liters of fatty tissue were suctioned out (up to over 20 L of pure fatty tissue in one operation). This is a strategy that no one would approve of today. However, these experiences and complications have shaped us in retrospect and influenced our current standard of care. Combined surgical and conservative treatment, as we perform it today, was not standard back then.

Surgical therapy (Fig. 3.11) has now emerged from the shadow of purely conservative treatment, and we have long since ceased to say that purely conservative treatment must be exhausted in order to initiate surgical therapy. It depends on the treatment goal, your wishes, and medical aspects.

Conservatively oriented clinics often don't leave a good hair on liposuction and lump all surgical concepts together, although both sides are noticeably working to

Fig. 3.11 Performing liposuction using the waterjet-assisted technique

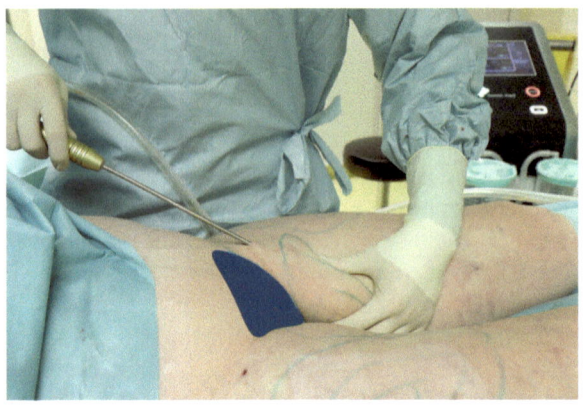

overcome the hurdles and understand and acknowledge each other's concepts—apart from some lymphatic therapists who still believe that lifelong lymphatic drainage therapy is the golden path. At this point, we ask patients who hold this conviction to pause for a moment and reflect on how much they are benefiting from their manual therapy in the long term and whether compression is the right path for them.

Our treatment strategy of complex surgical treatment is completely unknown to many. Complex because liposuction as a surgical measure is one of many components that lead to success (Fig. 3.12).

Since we often make initial diagnoses and initiate conservative treatment initially (decisive for the insurance applications), we can estimate quite well how much success the conservative treatment brings according to our experience. After 6 months we evaluate our initiated treatment consisting of compression (formerly in combination with lymphatic drainage) and nutritional or exercise therapy. We have rarely seen long-term positive courses of conservative treatments. It should be mentioned that these results are observational and not from a blinded scientific study.

It is possible, of course, that many patients who have received purely conservative treatment externally do not find their way to us because they no longer have any complaints, and consequently only those who respond poorly to conservative treatment present to us. However, this contradicts the initial diagnostic treatment we perform. We have no other possible explanations for these observations. Certainly, we have also seen patients who have improved only by compression treatment and a change in their lifestyle, including diet. However, this is rather the exception than the rule.

▶   Lipedema is not curable by either conservative or surgical therapy.

We are now of the opinion that conservative therapy has its justification, but is not the only option. It should certainly not be exhausted for years, only to be replaced by surgical therapy. We often see a lasting effect with our concept of complex-surgical treatment. It is important for us to make an honest indication and to see who is suitable for surgical intervention and who is not.

Fig. 3.12 Liposuction as a building block of the treatment plant

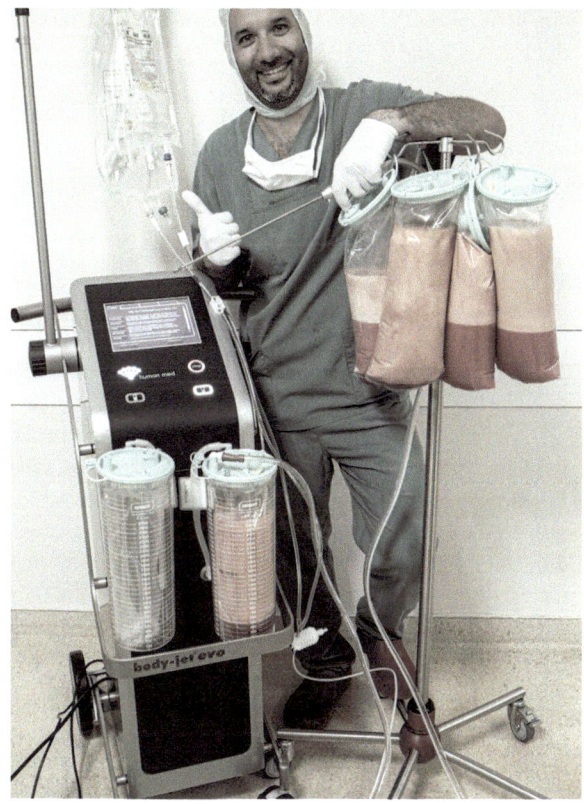

▶ We often see a lasting effect through our concept of complex surgical treatment.

If the accusation comes that surgeons naturally only want to operate, we have to face it and can—until science is ready—only give our experience and opinion based on it to the best of our knowledge and belief. Regardless of the treatment, our primary goal is to treat your pain. Other goals are to promote your mobility and to support you so that you can do again everything that you were no longer able to do due to the changes caused by lipedema—always with the best possible aesthetic result in mind.

Of course, we also want you to be satisfied with your external appearance and body contour. We always keep this aspect in mind during the surgical therapy of lipedema. This also means that we not only remove disturbing fatty tissue, but also treat any excess skin that may occur during large-volume liposuction. It does not make sense to suction out disturbing and painful fatty tissue from you, but then leave you to fend for yourself with excess and hanging skin. Unfortunately, this is exactly the problem we see very often, because many of the doctors who are not trained in plastic surgery do not offer tightening surgery. Therefore, tightening surgery is also an important selection criterion for choosing a plastic and aesthetic surgery specialist. You can find out more about how to find a suitable doctor in Chap. 5.

▶   Especially if you suffer from pronounced lipedema, you should look for a practitioner who also performs tightening surgery. Ask if their practitioner also performs thigh lifts and upper arm lifts. Ask to see results of these tightening surgeries.

A much advertised claim is that the previous need for lymphatic drainage after liposuction no longer exists. The first question to ask here, of course, is: Was lymphatic drainage actually necessary before? Probably rather not. So here professional providers of liposuction take up a previously unnecessary wrong treatment in order to advertise that it is no longer necessary afterwards.

Even if lipedema appears complex, it can be broken down into individual components. Therefore, liposuction makes absolute sense in many constellations. If liposuction is performed in our clinic, this is always done according to a previously prepared therapy plan—whether in the case of overweight patients with a change in diet and exercise therapy or in the case of morbid obesity with prior weight reduction through bariatric surgery. All measures are building blocks of our complex surgical treatment.

▶   In most cases, liposuction is only part of the lipedema treatment.

Liposuction can only be successful if all criteria for a successful treatment are met in advance. These include, among other things, a stable weight, the necessary compliance, well-controlled physical or psychological concomitant diseases, if present, and last but not least realistic expectations of the result.

3.5   The Individual Therapy Plan

Each of us is different. There is a huge variety of body shapes and equally different manifestations of lipedema. Therefore, we create an individual therapy plan for each affected person.

What does our complex surgical treatment for lipedema look like in detail? In the run-up, we often, but not necessarily, perform a purely conservative treatment for at least 6 months. This is mainly due to the fact that the health insurance companies require this procedure for an application for reimbursement. During this time, other underlying diseases should be excluded (e.g. venous disease). For the initial treatment, we recommend flat-knitted compression stockings of class 2. If there is confirmed edema in the sense of lipo-lymphedema, supportive manual lymphatic drainage may be useful.

If your parameters and body constitution speak for the existence of significant obesity (also taking into account the WHR and WHtR), the treatment of lipedema is always preceded by weight reduction. This means in 95% of massively overweight cases a metabolic intervention in the sense of gastrointestinal surgery in a specialized center for obese people. We cannot and do not want to use BMI values for patients with lipedema, but must decide on a case-by-case basis. There is certainly an indication for surgery if the BMI is clearly >40 kg/m^2. However, surgery is often indicated even if lipedema is not severe and the BMI is <40 kg/m^2, e.g., if concomitant diseases are present.

▶ An individual therapy plan tailored to you is necessary for optimal treatment.

For those affected with mild to moderate obesity and lipedema, regardless of its severity, we recommend a nutritional analysis and, if necessary, adjustment, as well as an activity-enhancing change in general lifestyle. This therapy plan is supplemented by a plan of surgical treatment.

For lipedema patients with a minor, moderate, or pronounced disproportion without a significant component of obesity, we recommend liposuction as the central surgical component of complex surgical treatment. We also include in this group patients who have previously treated their obesity with weight reduction.

The last component of the complex-surgical treatment is the inclusion in the therapy plan of the skin-soft tissue excesses that in some cases become apparent after liposuction. The treatment of these skin-soft tissue excesses is carried out by means of adapted tightening operations. These are always carried out at the expense of the statutory health insurance if a physical disfigurement or changes with a pathological value occur. These are, for example, repeated infections and chronic chafing in the area of skin overlaps. Restrictions on movement caused by the excess skin are also included.

▶ The complex-surgical treatment plan consists of three main pillars:
▶ Weight reduction or stabilization if necessary (conservative or surgical).
▶ Liposuctions.
▶ Tissue tightening if needed.

The sequence of treatment steps always includes weight stabilization as the first step. At the same time, we recommend adjusting and optimizing any accompanying psychological or physical illnesses. The consistent change of diet and lifestyle toward more activity can take place in accompanying programs. If there is a risk of relapse into old behavioral patterns, an accompanying behavioral therapy may have to be considered. If the pain is very severe, pain management therapy may be useful.

3.6   The Liposuction

3.6.1   General Information

Suck off fat? You've probably heard something about this before. The principle of liposuction is relatively easy to explain: the subcutaneous fatty tissue is suctioned off in a controlled manner through a small incision in the skin, which is approx. 5 mm long, using cannulas of different diameters (Fig. 3.13). Many also use the term "liposuction" as a synonym for liposuction, which was introduced by the English "liposuction."

The first reports of attempts at liposuction are attributed to the Frenchman Charles Dujarrier. Unfortunately, it was really just an "attempt." Dujarrier attempted to remove fatty tissue from a dancer's legs using sharp cannulas. The endeavor was unsuccessful and resulted in a leg amputation after injury to a major blood vessel. It was Joseph Schrudde who conducted further experiments with sharp instruments and a suction device in the 1960s and 1970s. In 1976, two Americans, Arpad and Giorgio Fischer, published for the first time a concept of suction with a blunt cannula.

Finally, it was Yves-Gerard Illouz who promoted the use of a liposuction fluid to prepare the fat tissue. This approach was not yet mature at that time. For a long time, developments around liposuction stagnated until J. Klein set a new milestone in 1987 by "inventing" tumescent anesthesia. This tumescent anesthesia, which we will also refer to in simplified terms as "special saline solution," solved the major problem of bleeding tendency during the operation. Further innovations were the further development of cannulas and technical devices, which are still used today for liposuction.

Liposuction can be performed as a stand-alone procedure, as in lipedema, or as purely aesthetic liposuction or as a partial step in combination with another operation. A distinction is made as to whether liposuction is used only as a fine contouring procedure or as an actual volume reduction in combination with contouring, which is often performed for lipedema. In fine contouring, liposuction is used only to create smooth transitions and definition. A classic example of this is abdominoplasty and breast lift, where liposuction is often used only for the transitional regions. The situation is different with liposuction as a stand-alone procedure: here, the aim is usually to uniformly remove as much volume as possible while at the same time shaping a contour.

Fig. 3.13 Insertion for performing liposuction

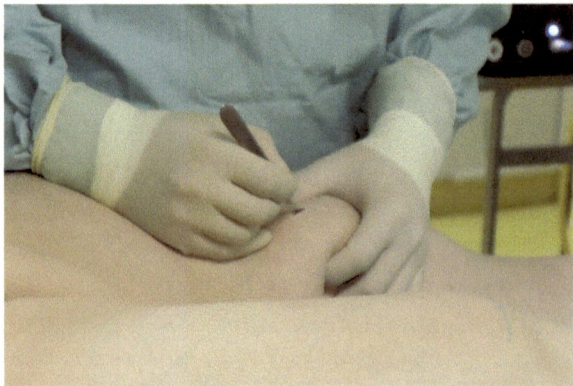

3.6.2   Techniques and Shapes

In order to perform liposuction, it is necessary to prepare the fatty tissue for this suction. This is done by introducing a special saline solution into the tissue. This special saline solution (also known as tumescent solution in technical jargon) consists of saline, a local anesthetic for pain suppression, adrenaline, and a buffer (solution for balancing the acid-base balance in the tissue; Fig. 3.14). Due to the local anesthetic of the solution, liposuction can be performed very well only with the special saline solution without general anesthesia.

By introducing the special saline solution, three main effects are achieved:

1. Local anesthesia eliminates the sensation of pain.
2. The adrenaline in the solution causes blood vessels to constrict, resulting in much less bleeding into the tissue.
3. Flushing the fat tissue with this solution loosens it up and prepares it for liposuction.

Fig. 3.14 Preparing the tumescent solution

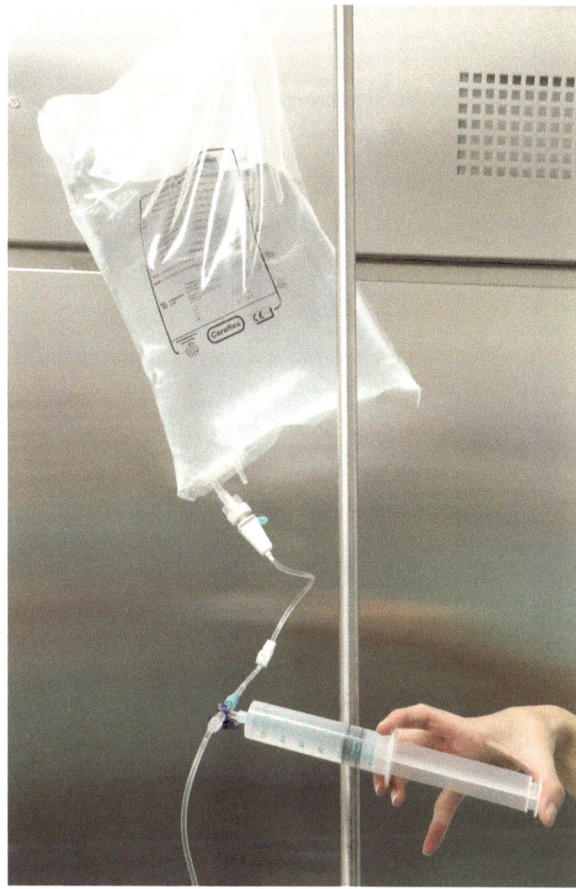

Depending on how much special saline solution (amount in ml) is introduced into the fatty tissue, the common suction methods are also called wet ("wet"), super wet ("super wet"), and tumescent methods. The tumescent and super-wet methods introduce a lot of fluid into the tissue. Just to understand the quantities: The super-wet method puts about as much special saline solution into the body as fat tissue is to be removed (1:1). The situation is different with the tumescent method. Here, two to three times as much fluid is brought into the tissue as fatty tissue is to be removed. We recommend the tumescent or super-wet method, but each surgeon has his or her own preference.

The Dry technique, which completely avoids the use of tumescent solution, is not recommended. This technique causes severe tissue trauma and often leads to unsightly dents and ripples. Moreover, uncontrolled bleeding and very severe scarring may occur.

We recommend the classic wet method, which represents a good middle ground. With this method, not too much liquid is introduced and an assessment of the possible result is still possible.

▶ We recommend liposuction with the tumescent or super-wet method and strongly advise against dry liposuction without fluid (dry method).

Technically apparatively we distinguish different systems with which we can perform liposuction. We distinguish classic liposuction from water jet–assisted liposuction (WAL), power or vibration assisted liposuction (PAL), ultrasound liposuction, laser liposuction, and many others, the list of which would go beyond the scope of this article. However, we would like to go into more detail about some of the techniques mentioned.

As mentioned, all techniques involve loosening of the fatty tissue via the special saline solution (tumescent solution). From a scientific point of view, none of the techniques described below can be said to be superior. Rather, each practitioner has his or her own personal technique. With regard to the possible forms of anesthesia, the methods do not differ. All of them are possible in a local partial or general anesthesia. We will come to the forms of anesthesia later on.

In our clinic, most of the techniques listed below are used with the various systems. Due to the diverse systems available, an individual adaptation to the respective patient can be made.

Fig. 3.15 Different cannula of different systems

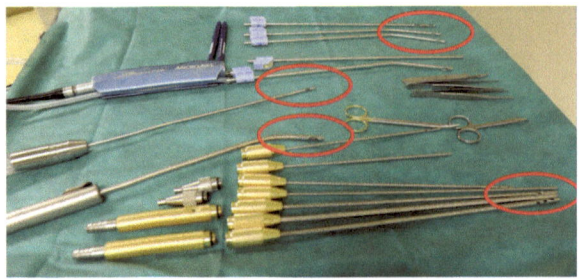

▶ From our point of view, the method or system of liposuction is secondary. More important are the training and experience of the surgeon.

For each system, there are different cannulas with which the fat is aspirated (Fig. 3.15). We distinguish between cannulas with small diameters of 2–3 mm and very large-lumen cannulas with 5–6 mm. We also distinguish between cannulas with many or few openings and straight from curved cannulas. Some cannulas are more rigid than others are slightly more flexible. Another decisive difference is the sharpness of the holes, so some cannulas have very sharp holes and can thus almost cut and others are very blunt.

In the case of large-volume liposuction, large-lumen cannulas tend to be used in the operation at the beginning, and thinner cannulas are then used as the operation progresses. The thinner cannulas are thus used more for definition and fine contouring.

Before we discuss the different systems, let's briefly look at the manual technique. Many differentiate between purely aesthetic liposuction and liposuction for lipedema in terms of manual technique. The distinction should be made on the basis of lymphatic vessel sparing and non-lymphatic vessel sparing. It is said that in lipedema liposuction is performed only parallel to the lymphatic vessels and in aesthetic liposuction also in a so-called criss-cross technique.

In the initial chapters, we talked about the anatomy of lymphatic vessels. Let us now imagine a moving liposuction cannula in close proximity to a lymphatic vessel. If we suction parallel to the lymphatic vessels, they can certainly be injured less quickly than if we perform liposuction at right angles to the lymphatic vessels. We view the entire discussion about parallel and nonparallel suctioning to the lymphatic vessels in aesthetic procedures and in lipedema as critical. In our opinion, the lymphatic vessels must always be handled gently and considerately, regardless of whether lipedema is involved or not. It is not so much a question of the direction of suction, but rather how sharp the cannulas are (by this we mean the sharpness of the holes) that are used. Sharp cannulas cut the tissue and thus also lymphatic vessels. It is therefore important to avoid sharp cannulas.

Finally, let's talk about negative pressure during liposuction. All techniques require negative pressure to suction off the fat cells. The interaction of negative pressure, cannula, and cannula sharpness is particularly important. The more negative the negative pressure, the more aggressively the fat tissue is suctioned out. Liposuction is performed at −100 to −1000 mbar. Relatively little fatty tissue is suctioned at −100 mbar and a great deal at −1000 mbar. But the negative pressure does not only have an effect on the fat cells; of course, it also has an effect on the surrounding tissue. If we work with a very negative pressure, injury to the surrounding tissue is more likely, because the tissue is sucked in more. So if we change one component (negative pressure, cannula holes, cannula sharpness), it will affect the entire liposuction procedure. Here it is important to achieve a harmonious interaction of all components.

Classic Liposuction

In classic liposuction, rigid, straight, or curved cannulas are used (Fig. 3.16). It is the classic image as we know it from television. Apart from a system that creates suction, no other aids are used.

Classic liposuction still has its justification today. It works perfectly and is the most frequently used method worldwide. However, it is possible to make life much easier for the surgeon by using machine support, e.g., with the systems presented below (Fig. 3.17). Nevertheless, we continue to use classical liposuction, especially for small, circumscribed liposuctions to obtain fat tissue for autologous fat transplantation.

The disadvantage of classic liposuction is that we see significant fibrosis of the fatty tissue, especially in advanced courses. The more advanced fibrosis is, the more "troublesome" liposuction is. The same is aggravated after liposuction, the internal fibrosis and scarring continue to increase. Once an area has been liposuctioned, it is difficult to perform a second liposuction in that area. Therefore, various devices have been established to "simplify" liposuction. In the following, we will discuss some of these supporting devices.

Fig. 3.16 Classic cannulas for liposuction

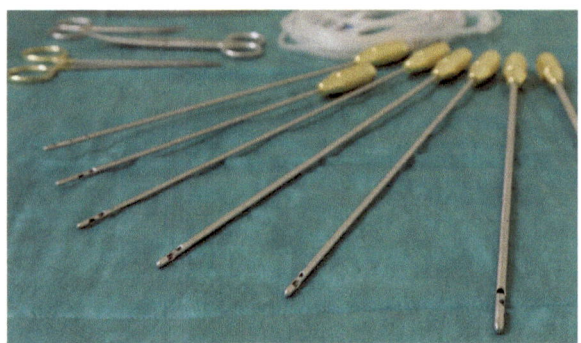

Fig. 3.17 WAL + PAL + classic liposuction

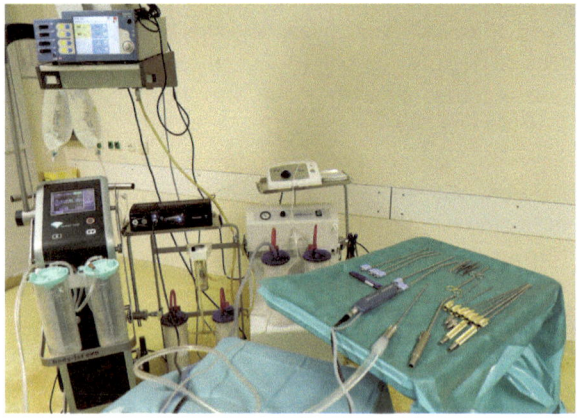

Water Jet Assisted Liposuction

Water jet–assisted liposuction is also called Bodyjet liposuction (from the name of the device that is used) or high-pressure water jet liposuction. WAL has been around for over 10 years, and it has found its permanent place in liposuction procedures. In WAL, a special device called a bodyjet is used. The special thing about this is that in this form of liposuction a water jet continuously assists (assists) the liposuction, hence the name. The liposuction is performed through a double-lumen cannula. Liposuction is performed via the outer large-lumen portion, while the smaller inner portion of the cannula is used for simultaneous injection of tumescent solution (Fig. 3.18).

In all forms of liposuction, the special saline solution is introduced into the fatty tissue at the beginning of liposuction, usually with quite a large volume (tumescent or super-wet method). This is different in the WAL method. Here, although tumescent solution is also infiltrated at the beginning of liposuction, it is in a much smaller volume, which is only sufficient for anesthesia and initial preparation of the fat tissue, as the continuous water jet makes its own contribution to further anesthesia and fat cell release during liposuction. This gives a small advantage to aesthetic liposuction procedures where little fat tissue is present and consequently little is to be suctioned. The inexperienced surgeon can better judge the contours if not too much tumescent solution has been infiltrated.

One advantage of WAL is the simultaneous flushing out of the fat cells during liposuction. This is supposed to be gentler and less traumatic for the tissue, but also for the triggered fat cells. In the case of autologous fat transplantation, this method is preferred because fewer stem cells are to be destroyed than with other methods. We also use WAL in addition to PAL for second or third liposuction when areas have already been liposuctioned. Many refer to WAL as new and innovative, which it is not. In our opinion, the WAL method has been replaced by the PAL method in many areas.

▶   The WAL method is one of our standard methods of liposuction, along with PAL and classic liposuction.

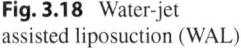
Fig. 3.18 Water-jet assisted liposuction (WAL)

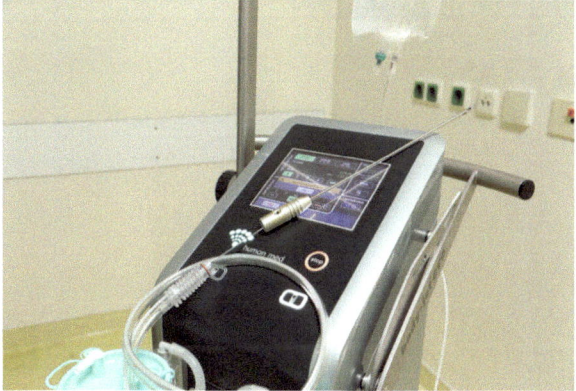

Power-Assisted Liposuction

Vibration-assisted liposuction is also known as power-assisted liposuction or PAL. The word "power" already gives a lot away. The system does indeed have "power" in it and is one of my personal favorites among liposuction systems.

Unlike the Bodyjet, which is produced by only one company for WAL, there are significantly more manufacturers offering a PAL system in the power-assisted systems segment. The main difference to waterjet-assisted liposuction is that the cannulas of the PAL can either only infiltrate or only suction, but not both at the same time. Consequently, with this technique, it is necessary to infiltrate first and then suction in a very classic way.

The principle behind PAL is to release the fat cells from the tissue complex with vibrational energy. The surgeon holds a handpiece with a "motor" in his hand that triggers vibrations (Fig. 3.19). Different cannulas can then be attached to this handpiece. The vibration generated, although somewhat more powerful, is similar to that of the well-known ultrasonic vibration toothbrushes. The fat cells are aspirated simultaneously with the release.

The PAL method is gentle on tissue and particularly suitable for large-volume liposuction. But fine contouring can also be performed very well with the PAL method. I personally prefer the PAL method to most other methods for first, second, and third liposuctions. It is also very well suited for autologous fat transplants and offers the best results in our hands with WAL. In Fig. 3.19 you can see a PAL system for liposuction.

▶   PAL suction is one of the most suitable techniques for the treatment of lipedema.

Ultrasound Assisted Liposuction

Ultrasound-assisted liposuction (UAL)is also a long-established method that has found some enthusiasts. It was established in Europe in the 1990s and is not widely used. It uses low-energy ultrasound, and liposuction is performed over 3 substeps. First is the infiltration of the tumescent solution, the second step is the release of the

Fig. 3.19 Handle (motor) of power-assisted liposuction

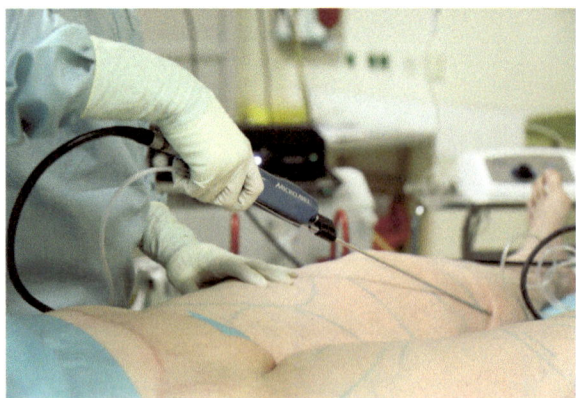

fat cells from the connective tissue complex via the ultrasound probe, and finally, in the third and final step, the detached fat cells are suctioned out. Of course, nerves, blood vessels, and skin remain unharmed during ultrasound-assisted liposuction. Some colleagues consider this form of liposuction less suitable for autologous fat grafting, although clinical studies show that fat tissue suctioned by UAL can also be used for autologous fat grafting.

Manufacturers of UAL devices see a great advantage of UAL in body contouringor body sculpting. In this case, the body is particularly defined during suction, such as a six pack on the abdomen, which is then simulated by fat. But all other methods can also be used very well for body sculpting; it is just a question of the method.

Laser-Assisted Liposuction
In laser-assisted liposuction, the fat cells are destroyed by a laser that simultaneously spares the surrounding connective tissue. The heat generated by the laser stimulates collagen synthesis in the connective tissue, which should lead to tissue shrinkage and associated tightening effect.

Especially this method requires an experienced surgeon. In the past years, we have seen some patients with unsightly dents and skin defects after burns caused by such laser liposuction. In our opinion, the propagated tissue shrinkage by the laser can also be achieved by using other techniques with specific cannulas or by using tightening devices (Sect. 4.2). This feature of laser liposuction should therefore not be the decisive selection criterion for this form of liposuction. If you are interested in laser liposuction, seek out a truly experienced surgeon who has been performing laser liposuction for some time. The results are usually the same with skilled surgeons regardless of the technique used.

3.6.3   Liposuction Volume

One of the questions we are most frequently asked, apart from the technique used, is the maximum number of liters of fatty tissue we can aspirate in one operation (Fig. 3.20). In order to answer this question in a comprehensible way, we must first take a closer look at the "liter figure."

As already explained, before liposuction, a special saline solution (tumescent solution) is introduced into the tissue to prepare the fatty tissue for liposuction. During liposuction, fat cells and portions of the tumescent solution are suctioned out. The remainder of the tumescent solution is eventually absorbed by the body (Fig. 3.21). The "suction bag" now contains the so-called lipoaspirate as a fat-tumescent solution mixture.

▶   The lipoaspirate is a mixture of liquid and fatty tissue.

Quantity Specification
There are two ways of specifying the quantity. Either the total amount of lipoaspirate or the pure fat amount is indicated. If you want to specify the pure amount of

Fig. 3.20 Lipoaspirate after waterjet-assisted liposuction

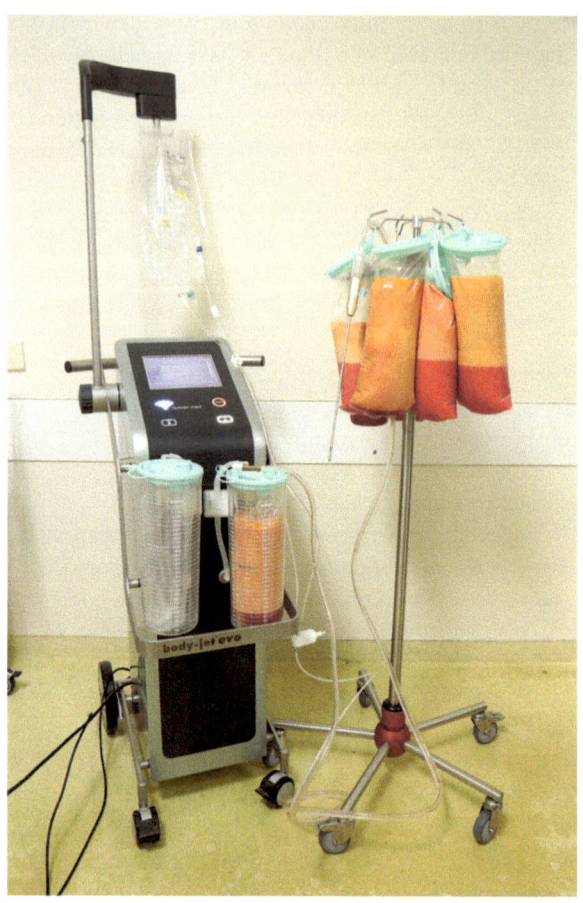

Principle of liposuction

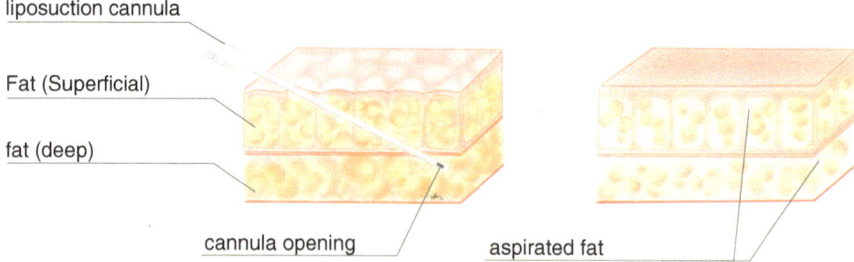

liposuction cannula

Fat (Superficial)

fat (deep)

cannula opening

aspirated fat

Fig. 3.21 Principle of liposuction

fat, you must allow time for the lipoaspirate to settle from the water. Since fat has a lower density than water, the fat settles in the upper phase and water in the lower phase. Thus, the pure amount of fat tissue can be indicated. But even then, there is still a certain amount of fluid between the fat cells, although not much. The longer you give the lipoaspirate time, the more accurate the pure adipose tissue quantity can be indicated.

Unfortunately, there is no standard for specifying the volumes aspirated. It is best to ask your surgeon whether the figure is for pure adipose tissue or for lipoaspirate (fat + liquid), so that you know how to interpret the figures.

Depending on which method is used for liposuction and how small or large the cannulas are, the total amount of liposuction varies. Liposuction with very small cannulas (WAL or PAL) results in a lower amount of pure fat tissue than with large-lumen cannulas (classic liposuction). It is most likely due to the fact that the cells are separated more and no conglomerates are suctioned, which are more condensed.

We have often seen that only the total volume is given in surgery reports. The pure fat volume should always be stated so that it is comparable and others do not stand out with a misleading "I suction more." We always state our liposuction volumes as pure fat volumes after an appropriate "settling time" of about 20 min.

▶   Liposuction volume should always be reported as fat-only to ensure consistent documentation.

In Fig. 3.22, we see different lipoaspirates with different proportions of fatty and aqueous phase. Aspirated quantities of fatty tissue vary from a few milliliters

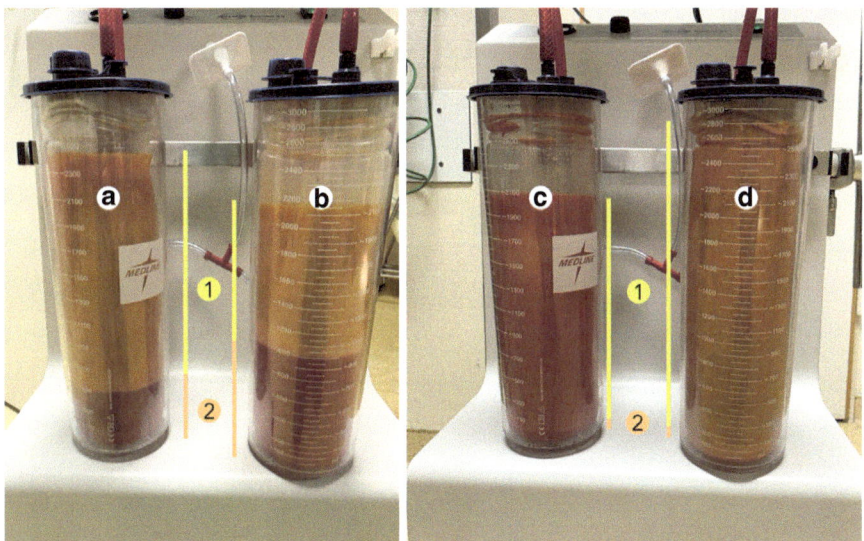

Fig. 3.22 Different lipoaspirates. A, B fat phase (1) and water phase (2); C, D almost exclusively pure fat tissue (without 1) and only low water phase (2)

(Fig. 3.23), such as in cosmetic procedures on the face (neck or cheek suction) or for use as a filler for autologous fat transplants for wrinkle treatment, to over 10 L of pure fat in so-called megaliposuctions. The term megaliposuction is not defined and is very vague. Many understand a megaliposuction as a total lipoaspirate quantity (fat and liquid) of more than 5 L. For us, megaliposuctions are defined as a suctioned, pure fat quantity of more than 10 L.

Safe Suction Volume

The scientific landscape is divided on the safety of liposuction. In America, pure fat amounts of 3–5% of one's own body weight are indicated as safe. In Europe, scientific papers show a safe amount of suction of 8–10% of one's own body weight.

This means that for a body weight of 80 kg, liposuction of 3% of body weight results in a pure amount of fatty tissue of 2.4 L, and for a suction amount of 10% of body weight, 8 L. Thus, quite a large variable is shown when it comes to the amount of fat tissue suctioned. Table 3.3 shows an example of the different quantities depending on body weight.

▶   There is no consensus on how much fat tissue should be suctioned out
     in a low-risk surgery.

How do such different statements regarding the maximum suction volume come about? This is simply a matter of safety and risk minimization. In general, the less fatty tissue that is aspirated, the lower the risk. We would like to go into this problem in a little more detail.

Fig. 3.23 Approximately 20 mL of fat for autologous fat grafting

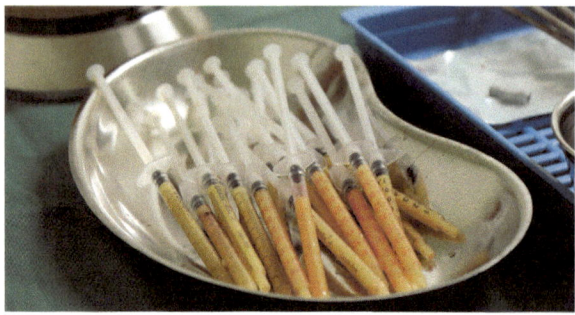

Table 3.3 Safe fat aspirate by aspiration amount and body weight

Body weight (kg)	3% Fat aspirate (L)	5% Fat aspirate (L)	8% Fat aspirate (L)	10% Fat aspirate (L)
70	2.1	3.5	5.6	7.0
80	2.4	4.0	6.4	8.0
90	2.7	4.5	7.2	9.0
100	3.0	5.0	8.0	10.0
110	3.3	5.5	8.8	11.0

Aspect Tumescent Solution

The more volume is to be suctioned, the more tumescent solution is introduced into the tissue. The special saline solution often contains lidocaine as a local anesthetic. Above a certain concentration, this can lead to an oxygen deficiency in the body, which is due to the fact that the drug alters (oxidizes) the red blood pigment "hemoglobin," resulting in so-called methemoglobin. Due to its higher binding power to oxygen, it deprives it from hemoglobin, and there is an oxygen deficiency in our body. Symptoms are the classic signs such as headache, fatigue, shortness of breath, lethargy, and blue discoloration of the skin and mucous membrane.

We and many other practitioners therefore resort to an alternative local anesthetic to avoid this problem. Others do not use a local anesthetic at all and only perform the treatments under general anesthesia and without any addition of local anesthetics. We feel that the local anesthetic in the tumescent solution is a good and sensible pain treatment for the first hours after the operation. Therefore, in our opinion, a certain amount of local anesthetic should always be used to ensure pain relief after surgery.

Aspect Dilution

During liposuction, the introduction of the tumescent solution, which is absorbed by the body in large proportions, results in a dilution effect of the blood. Blood consists of about half liquid blood plasma and half blood cells or blood corpuscles. The percentage of blood cells in relation to the total blood volume is called hematocrit. Since the red blood cells, the so-called erythrocytes, make up approx. 99% of the blood cells and ensure oxygen transport in the body, a low hematocrit value indicates a low proportion of red blood cells and thus a low oxygen transport capacity (Fig. 3.24). Consequences of a too low hematocrit can be dizziness,

Hematocrit

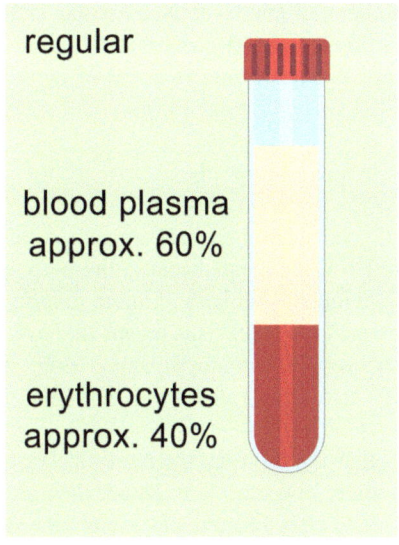
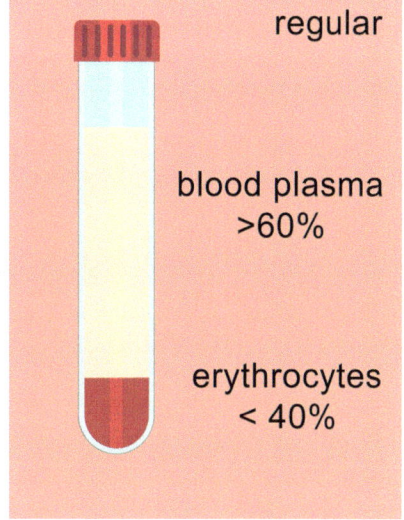

Fig. 3.24 Blood composition (hematocrit)

nausea, pallor, circulatory weakness, lack of strength, loss of appetite, malaise, and headache.

▶   The hematocrit value indicates the proportion of red blood cells in the total blood volume. The normal value for women is a hematocrit of 37–45%.

▶   If there is too much fluid or too few red blood cells in the blood, this is called dilution. Dilution is indicated by a lowered hematocrit value (HK or Hkt value).

Aspect Bleeding
Of course, bleeding occurs in any surgery, both during and after the procedure. Bleeding has historically always been the main problem with liposuction. They have limited liposuction for a very long time. The larger the procedure, the higher the risk of bleeding becomes. In surgery with a proper skin incision, you would see the source of bleeding and perform hemostasis via cauterization of the blood vessels. However, this is not possible with liposuction because we operate with long cannulas through a small incision of about 5 mm. Therefore, the "adrenaline" in the special saline solution is indispensable. It acts on the blood vessels and causes them to contract. This has two effects: First, the small blood vessels close their lumen (the opening where blood flows through). Second, the blood vessels take up less space in the tissue, and injury with the suction cannulas is reduced. We know pretty much when and how well the epinephrine is working, because as soon as the epinephrine kicks in, the skin turns completely white as a sign of decreased blood flow, also known as the blanching effect (whitening) in medical jargon. But also during the operation we can see how the lipoaspirate looks in the tube. If it is golden yellow, then there is little to no blood mixed in. If it is red or reddish, there is more blood mixed in with the lipoaspirate. Nevertheless, there is always some blood loss.

Blood loss is accompanied by a drop in the hemoglobin level. Hemoglobin (Hb) is the red blood pigment and a protein of red blood cells (erythrocytes). The most important task of hemoglobin is the transport of oxygen and removal of carbon dioxide in the blood.

▶   Blood loss is accompanied by a drop in hemoglobin levels.

The hemoglobin value depends on age and gender. Women have a normal value range of 12–16 g/dL. If bleeding occurs, the Hb value drops because the body is unable to produce new red blood cells quickly enough. Similarly, dilution (overhydration with tumescent solution) leads to a lowered Hb level. This means that overhydration with tumescent solution causes a drop in hematocrit and a drop in hemoglobin, and the drop in hemoglobin is also aggravated by a real loss of erythrocytes.

Thus, the greater the blood loss and the higher the dilution, the more likely are reduced performance, shortness of breath (initially only during exertion, then also at rest), palpitations and ringing in the ears, pale skin and mucous membrane. If blood loss is too great, a blood transfusion must be given. In the worst case, one can bleed to death from it.

How much blood you actually lose depends on various factors. Physical factors, technical aspects, and surgical factors. Physical factors include how good one's blood clotting is, how fit and well one's body works, whether one suffers from high blood pressure, and whether there is any family history of clotting disorders (which often do not warrant liposuction), etc. Like anyone who focuses on liposuction, we have our own technique. Depending on whether we operate under general or local anesthesia, we use an adapted composition of tumescent solution. Especially in the case of high-volume liposuction, we have modified it to further reduce the complications mentioned, such as dilution, side effects of local anesthetics, and bleeding.

Time Expenditure
According to the effort required, the time needed for liposuction varies from 30 min to over 4 h. At the same time, liposuction in a very slim lady who is undergoing treatment for purely aesthetic reasons or for atypical lipedema can take much longer than a 10-L megaliposuction, with a suctioned pure fat volume of 2–3 L. It depends on the actual effort and how much care the region needs at the moment of treatment. For example, the lower leg region is considered time-consuming, the upper back region is considered difficult to perform and bloody compared to other regions (there are more powerful blood vessels in this region). Thus, each region has its own characteristics, which is also reflected as another factor on the aspect of time. Recent studies show that the surgical risk of complications increases with the duration of surgery. For most liposuction procedures we need at least 2 h of pure operation time with quite a lot of experience, but often 2.5–3 h, sometimes even longer. With sufficient experience, the pure operation time can be kept relatively short and effective. Very often liposuction is performed not only by one surgeon, but by a whole team. A well-coordinated team therefore brings advantages here. Do not compare your liposuctioned fat amounts with others, as the conditions are different and the time required differs depending on the region and the patient. Liposuction of the hips is difficult to compare with liposuction of the lower legs.

Outpatient–Inpatient?
Liposuction we generally perform on an outpatient basis up to a volume of 3–4 L. Many colleagues, especially those who operate in the practice, handle this somewhat differently. In some cases, they aspirate more volume and maintain a follow-up period of at least 12 h before discharge. There are certainly many ways to combine safety and patient comfort here. Our experience has shown that inpatient treatment for larger volumes has many advantages. The biggest advantage is that you can be monitored clinically (see how you are doing) and accordingly you can be supported in all your needs. There can also be infusion treatments and checks on blood values. Often you will lose fluid through the small incisions for liposuction afterwards, which is often uncomfortable at home. If you remain in the clinic, you can leave the leaking tumescent solution in the hospital without having to deal with it at home. If complications arise, someone will be there to help you. Those affected

say it is relaxing when you don't feel pressure to go home right after surgery. Likewise, follow-up is simplified during the first few days. We will see you every day without you having to be brought to or picked up from an office. Thus, we recommend to treat liposuction from 3 to 4 L inpatient for one night. The more voluminous the liposuction is, the longer a stay should be planned, as the physical adjustment reactions then usually take a little longer. For liposuction of 8 L or more of pure fat, we recommend a stay of 2–3 days. From 10 L it should be 3 days or longer. It should be pointed out again that we are talking about pure lipoaspirate quantities.

▶   For liposuction from 3 to 4 L, patients should stay in the hospital for at
    least 12 h.

3.7 Conclusion

In summary, we consider the discussion of maximum liposuction amounts to be difficult, as many factors must be taken into account. Experience with different techniques over a long time is also valuable here. When we say that we often suction fat volumes of much more than 10 L, it does not mean that everyone can do it on everyone. It depends on the overall constellation. We think that a large volume liposuction in a specialized center is associated with a lower risk than a "smaller liposuction" in untrained hands.

From our experience, we can say that about 10% of liposuctions are performed with a volume below 4 L of pure fat. In 50% of the patients, liposuction is performed with 4–8 L and in 40% of the cases, liposuction is performed with more than 8 L of pure fat volume.

▶   The most common amounts aspirated for lipedema settle between 4 and
    8 L of pure fat per surgery.
▶   Caution. Do not allow yourself to be "recruited" by colleagues with
    statements such as: "With us, there is no post-operative bleeding or
    hemorrhaging" or "Surgery without Hb drop." These statements are not
    serious. Liposuction is always associated with risks.

3.7.1 Requirements and Preparations

The following tips and information apply in principle to all liposuction procedures. Nevertheless, it should be noted that, for example, liposuction with 500 mL of suctioned fat on the abdomen has both a completely different course and different risk potential than liposuction of 12 L of pure fat on the legs. A very small liposuction will have almost no impact on your well-being. You will pretty much certainly not have any dizziness, nor will you have any major bruising or significant blood loss. On the other hand, with very extensive liposuction, the wound areas created are much larger. The anesthesia time is longer and the risk for complications is higher. Also, your recovery time after the procedure will be longer than after small, circumscribed liposuction. If your tissue is very fibrotic (connective tissue remodeling), liposuction is often more traumatic.

If you have morbid obesity and the treatment concept intends a combined treatment of obesity and lipedema, the obesity is usually treated first, by whatever options. Before the liposuction procedures, it would be helpful to reach the targeted weight as much as possible. Optimal would be a stable target weight for at least 6 months, better 1 year. This is certainly not a normal weight, as the lipedema component will not have disappeared.

Even if weight loss fails, it does not mean that all options have been exhausted or that liposuction per se is not possible. A solution approach can be found for you. If you do not suffer from severe obesity, the issue is not relevant for you.

For every operation, it is important to create the best possible starting conditions for an uncomplicated procedure and the subsequent healing process. All secondary diseases should be optimally controlled. If you suffer from secondary diseases, ask your attending physician how he or she assesses the condition of your secondary diseases and whether there are possibilities for further optimization. An example here would be a blood sugar disease (diabetes) and high blood pressure.

No matter what body constitution you have: Exercise regularly and activate your body metabolism through physical activity. This will strengthen your heart and circulatory system in the long term. It is the same with your muscle balance. A healthy muscle balance for the phase during and after the operation is helpful. This allows the body to process the operation better, and the recovery phase after the operation is significantly shortened. In addition, the overall tissue perfusion is much better in physically fit people than in nonathletic ones. You can thus significantly reduce the risk of complications through your own initiative. Unfortunately, many people who are about to have an operation think: "Sport? That's too late for me now. " Be told that it is never too late for that. Even if you start exercising two to three times a week only 8 or 6 weeks before surgery, it will have a positive effect on your treatment and psyche.

▶ Before surgery, make sure to adjust all secondary diseases in the best possible way. Try to make your body fit for the operation by exercising.

We have already discussed the topic of nutrition, and a balanced and healthy diet with an adequate supply of proteins, unsaturated fats, and important trace elements as well as vitamins is indispensable for a balanced metabolism in connection with an upcoming operation.

Smoking should be absolutely stopped before surgery, especially before liposuction! Smokers have much higher risks for the operation itself, but also for the course after the operation. It has been proven that smokers require higher doses of anesthetics and painkillers. Compared to nonsmokers, smokers have about six times the risk of pulmonary circulation complications after surgery. Examples would include pulmonary embolism or pneumonia. After surgery, smokers have about a three- to sixfold higher risk of wound healing problems and wound infections. The risk of thrombosis is also substantially increased.

Smokers suffer more often from diseases triggered by tobacco consumption such as cardiovascular diseases, respiratory diseases (e.g. chronic obstructive pulmonary disease, asthma), diabetes, and many others. All these diseases have a negative effect on the course after liposuction. Especially in the combination of liposuction plus smoking, the mentioned risk of thrombosis is a problem. Stopping smoking, the earlier the better, always has a positive effect on the operation, the recovery period, and the success of the operation (Fig. 3.25).

The immune system regenerates already within 4–6 weeks. Bronchial secretions and lungs recover after 6–8 weeks. Wound healing disorders occur less frequently if you stop smoking 4–6 weeks before surgery. If you do not manage to stop smoking, you should at least radically reduce your tobacco consumption. Even if the effect is not equal to smoking cessation and is less effective, at least a small risk reduction for surgery can be achieved by doing so.

Shortly before the operation (1–2 days) to give up the glow stick, unfortunately, no longer really brings much, but is still better than to continue to smoke, because the oxygen supply in the tissue is measurably better in comparison.

▶   Smoking cessation should definitely be attempted, preferably at least 8 weeks prior to surgery.

We already talked about the blood values and the hemoglobin level. In order for our body to produce functional red blood cells, it is necessary that our iron balance is balanced and that our iron reserves are well filled before an operation in order to be able to guarantee a problem-free new production of red blood cells. Now, is it a must to have a blood count check before any liposuction procedure and also check the iron storage levels? No, it is only a must if serious diseases are known. In some cases, we still recommend a blood count check, and in general there is nothing to be said against a check before a procedure if you want to be on the safe side.

If necessary, check your hemoglobin value (the hematocrit is lowered in anemia) and pay attention to the serum ferritin value. This value shows us the degree of filling of the iron store. If the iron balance is not balanced, it takes some time to

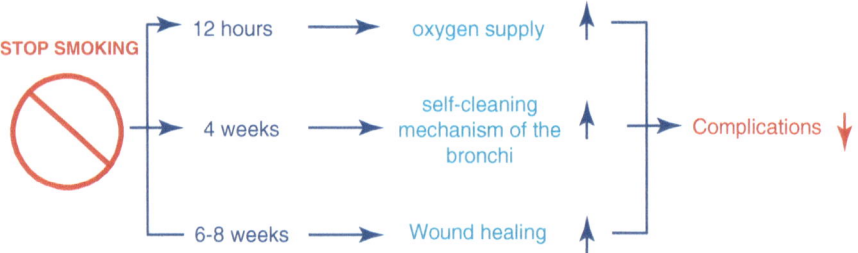

Fig. 3.25 Stop smoking

replenish the iron stores. In this case we recommend a long-term intake of iron supplements with appropriate control 4–8 weeks before surgery.

As an important building block for building and maintaining red blood cells, consumption and replenishment of the iron balance takes place. If an operation is performed and blood is lost naturally during the procedure, this automatically leads to increased iron consumption in order to produce new blood cells. This can lead to a relevant supply bottleneck of red blood cells and thus to surgery-related anemia. Therefore, it makes sense to pay attention to one's iron balance before surgery and to support it, for example, with iron-rich foods and, if necessary, with iron supplements from the health food store. We regularly recommend a herbal tonic with organically bound iron to our patients to prevent iron deficiency.

▶ Talk to your family doctor; if necessary, a blood count check is recommended before liposuction. We recommend preventing iron deficiency with a herbal tonic and organically bound iron.

At the time of surgery, it is important that you are healthy. You should not have a cold, diarrhea, or other illnesses. In case you fall ill before the operation, be fair to yourself and the surgeons and inform them in time. Otherwise, you are taking an incalculable risk, the consequences of which will affect you.

You should also not suffer from a local infection. Unfortunately, this occurs more often, especially with chronically rubbing together skin soft tissues as in stage III or with sufferers of acne inversa. If such an "infected pimple," open wound, or weeping redness is present shortly before or on the day of the operation, discuss it with your attending physician, even if the operation has to be postponed because of it. In principle, doctors do not do this to annoy you, but only for the sake of your health. An open wound or an acute abscess increases the risk of tissue infection, which does not have to be taken because this is not an emergency operation.

If you are taking a cortisone preparation due to a lung, rheumatic or other illness, it should be clarified in advance whether this can be discontinued. Cortisone can impair and delay wound healing. Discuss all your medications with us, including homeopathic and nonprescription medications. Avoid alcohol and any form of drugs prior to liposuction.

Do not take any blood-thinning medication before surgery. If you are dependent on blood thinning medication due to medical conditions, discuss this with your surgeon. We do not perform liposuction procedures while taking blood thinners. Some "headache pills" also contain blood thinners. Pay attention to this!

▶ Do not take any blood-thinning medications or homeopathic remedies before liposuction.

Please do not take homeopathic remedies before surgery. This also includes arnica. Although arnica has many positive properties, depending on the dosage, quite different effects result, and neither thrombosis through activation of clotting nor "blood thinning" in the sense of a tendency to bleed is desired. Therefore, the use of homeopathic remedies should be postponed until the days after surgery.

Before the procedure, already plan the time after the procedure. Do you have everything you need in the household? Is someone there for you after liposuction? Is everything ready so that you can easily get to things after the surgery? Do all the shopping in advance and maybe get some nice books or DVDs to pass the time.

Whether outpatient or inpatient treatment, organize reliable transportation home. We have seen patients come to the clinic in their own car after very complex aspirations and assume that they will be able to drive home again. However, this is not the case. You should not drive a vehicle either after extensive liposuctions or after circumscribed, small liposuctions.

To find out approximately how long you will be out of action, ask your practitioner in advance. Plan sufficient time for the downtime after the surgery. We give you a rough overview of downtime below, as we know it from our daily clinical routine. Of course, downtime is different for every patient and depends on how fit you are, how the surgery went, whether you tolerated the anesthesia well, etc. In addition, it depends on the profession and the activity in the profession. In Table 3.4, we have the total downtime (TAZ), which is the time you should really rest. After that, you can return to light exertion and simple activities, but you should refrain from sports or physically demanding work.

Despite this information, the courses can be very different. It is therefore better to plan a little more time than too little. If necessary, you should arrange with your employer for a sheltered job, that would certainly be a good option. If you have a family and children, this must also be organized.

Do you normally wear compression stockings and are affected by lipedema? If so, consistent compression should be worn before surgery, especially if you also suffer from an edema component.

▶ If you suffer from lipedema with an edema component, you should also wear your compression before liposuction.

Remember to change your compression supplies. Usually, the hospital will give you compression garments that are meant to be worn for the first period after surgery. Alternatively, you can wear your old compression garments after surgery. Get heparin ointment (60,000 IU) ahead of time to treat hematomas (bruises) after surgery. Rub the heparin ointment two to three times a day for 10–14 days.

After surgery, we recommend decongestant medications on a plant basis (homeopathics). For example, the active ingredient bromelanin has proven effective. This is

Table 3.4 Average total downtime (TAZ) after liposuction

Intervention	Number of exhausted liters	TAZ in days
Small outpatient liposuction	1–2	2–3
Suction on the legs and abdomen	Approx. 3	3–4
Medium suction	<5	7
Larger suction	>5	7–14
Very large extractions	>8	>21

available under various product names. Discuss its use with your doctor and obtain the product as a capsule from the pharmacy before the operation.

After liposuction, we recommend lymphatic drainage treatments. We will discuss the details in the course, but you can organize the appointments in advance.

If legs or arms are suctioned, then get enough pillows for elevation. Get old towels or pads for home to place under the suctioned areas, as fluid will continue to leak from the puncture sites for some time.

What you Should Consider Before Liposuction
1. Most importantly, you should go into liposuction in the best possible health and absolutely fit.
2. All underlying and secondary diseases such as diabetes, high blood pressure, etc. should be optimally controlled.
3. Do sports and activate your body metabolism. Your own initiative is required here.
4. Stop smoking! Smokers have significantly higher risks during surgery. Especially during liposuction, the risk of thrombosis is increased by tobacco consumption.
5. Make sure you eat a balanced diet.
6. If necessary, have your iron balance and hemoglobin checked. Serum ferritin and hemoglobin levels should be noted.
7. You must be healthy at the time of surgery. If you fall ill, please cancel the surgery in time.
8. Discuss all of your medications with your practitioner.
9. Cortisone preparations should be paused if possible. Consult your practitioner.
10. Do not take any blood-thinning medications before surgery, including homeopathic remedies.
11. Avoid alcohol and drugs before liposuction.
12. Before the procedure, already plan the time after the procedure. Do you have everything you need in the household? Is someone there for you after the operation?
13. Arrange transportation to surgery and return home.
14. Plan enough time off (vacation).
15. If you want to return to work early, take care of a gentle workplace.
16. If you have children, organize a support.
17. If you normally wear compression stockings, wear them consistently before surgery.
18. Think about alternate supply.
19. We recommend the use of heparin ointment after surgery 2 to 3 times a day.
20. We recommend the use of decongestant medications, such as bromelain.
21. Organize appointments for lymphatic drainage well in advance.
22. If legs or arms are suctioned, get enough pillows to elevate them.

Get old towels to place underneath at home. Fluid will continue to leak from the puncture sites for some time.

3.7.2   Liposuction Procedure

In summary, before liposuction, an introduction, examination, consultation, surgical explanation, and clarification of all administrative matters take place. The day before the surgery you should shower and put on fresh clothes. Do not put cream on your skin after showering, as we do our markings with a marking pen and it does not adhere well to creamed skin. Remove all earrings, piercings, and artificial nails. If you are having surgery in the pubic region, you should shave on the day of surgery. Arrive at surgery fasting, even if surgery is scheduled under a local anesthetic. Do not take any medications on your own that day.

Anesthesia
Liposuction can be performed in different anesthesia procedures. Most often, liposuction is performed under local anesthesia alone or under local anesthesia in combination with so-called analgesia (also known as twilight sleep). In the case of analgosedation, the patient's consciousness is dampened while being sedated and deprived of pain by medication. Analgesia does not involve intubation (insertion of a breathing tube into the airway) or mechanical ventilation. We prefer and recommend, whenever possible, local anesthesia in combination with twilight sleep. This combination is a very pleasant form of anesthesia for you, because you are virtually unaware of the whole procedure and yet do not have the risks of a general anesthetic. In addition to local anesthesia and the combination with twilight sleep, liposuction is often performed under general anesthesia.

▶   For lipedema, we usually recommend liposuction under general anesthesia.

When it comes to the topic of lipedema and high-volume liposuction, we very often advise general anesthesia. It is undisputed that with general anesthesia the risk is increased compared to analgosedation and local anesthesia. However, in recent years, these risks of general anesthesia have been reduced more and more. In contrast, comparatively more local anesthetic must be given for high-volume liposuction under local anesthesia than under general anesthesia. This also increases the risks described above. Weighing up the advantages and disadvantages as well as the risks, general anesthesia is absolutely preferable to analgesia and local anesthesia for high-volume liposuction.

Another aspect of liposuction is the positioning in the operation. Local anesthesia or analgosedation is an advantage for dynamic liposuction, where the positioning in the surgery often has to be changed (e.g., side-side-back position). A long prone position for liposuction of the backs of the legs or torso is not quite as comfortable under local anesthesia. Also, analgesia is rather impractical because the anesthesiologist does not have controlled access to the airways in this position. For this reason, we prefer to perform liposuction on lipedema patients under general anesthesia.

Procedure

Surely you are wondering how exactly liposuction is performed. Whether you are an outpatient or inpatient, you come to the clinic one day before or on the day of the operation. On the day of the operation, as with most plastic surgery operations, it begins with a drawing and surgical planning (Fig. 3.26).

This is also the right time to carry out photo documentation so that a before-and-after comparison is possible if required. Another nursing admission is made, and then in the course of the day we go to the operating room.

Depending on the treatment areas and the agreed form of anesthesia, either the induction of anesthesia and then the disinfection of your body takes place in the

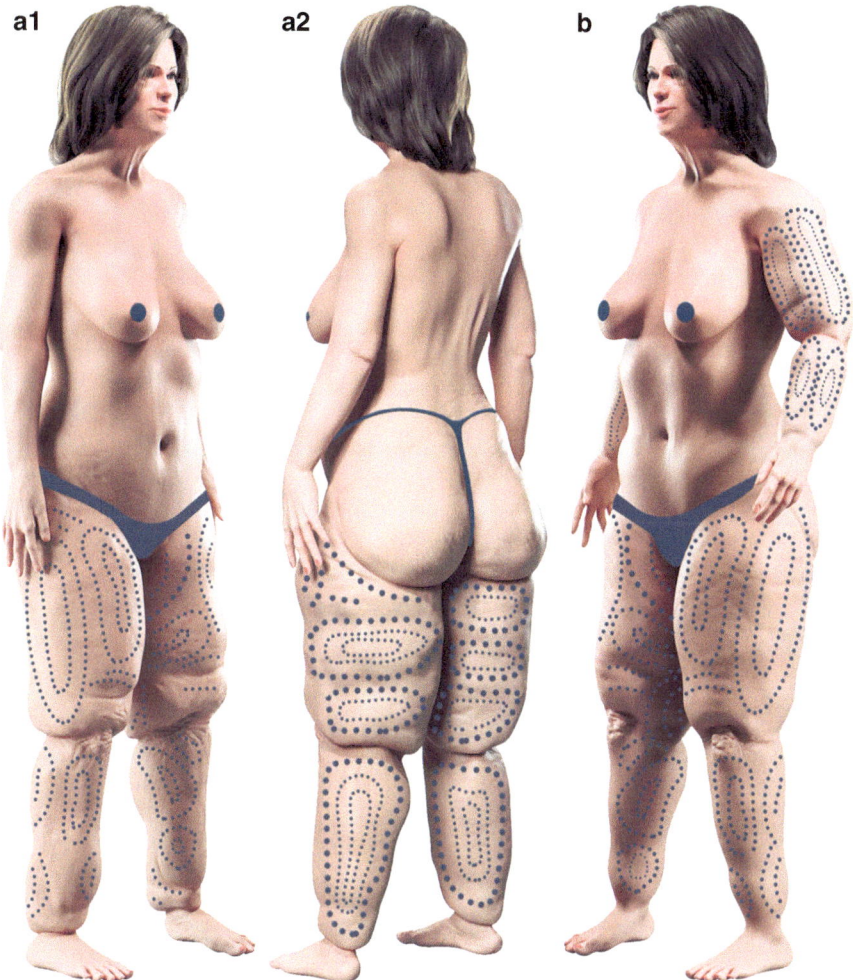

Fig. 3.26 Example drawing. A1, A2 Lipedema type III stage II; B Lipedema type IV stage II

operating room or the other way around. First, you are washed or disinfected while standing and then the anesthesia or local anesthesia is induced.

When and why does washing off (disinfection) take place while standing? Imagine that we are planning liposuction of the front and back of your legs (i.e., including the abdomen and back). The front and back of the legs as well as the abdomen and back are to be disinfected. If you are already asleep, this is possible, but unnecessarily complicated and time-consuming. Therefore, many liposuction procedures like to wash off while you are standing. Specifically, this means that you will be undressed and washed off or disinfected while standing before the anesthesia is administered. You will then lie down on an operating table covered with a sterile cloth. There you will be further covered with sterile drapes. Then the anesthesia is induced or local anesthesia is applied—depending on what has been agreed.

In some practices and clinics, local anesthesia is administered on a surgical couch using quite small needles. After the onset of the effect and before the surgery starts, washing off and covering are done. This is also a feasible way. We recommend performing liposuction in a proper operating room and not in an old converted living room or similar. Sterile conditions must be maintained.

▶   We recommend performing liposuction in a real operating room.

Let's assume a classic procedure: You come into the operating room, anesthesia is induced, and then the hips, legs, and arms are washed off and covered with sterile drapes. Then it's on to the operation itself. According to the agreement before the operation or according to the conditions in the operation, the approx. 5 mm large accesses for the introduction of the special saline solution (tumescent solution) are placed. After an exposure time of about 20 min, liposuction is started. In the first pass, the coarse fat pads are usually suctioned off, if they are present. This is done with relatively thick cannulas (5 and 6 mm). After this, fine contouring is performed in several passes (4- and 3-mm cannulas). Whether waterjet-assisted or power-assisted liposuction is performed is irrelevant for the procedure (Figs. 3.27 and 3.28). After sufficient thinning and ensuring symmetry, the skin incisions are closed by suturing at the end of the operation (Figs. 3.29 and 3.30).

Fig. 3.27 Setting for liposuction with WAL and PAL

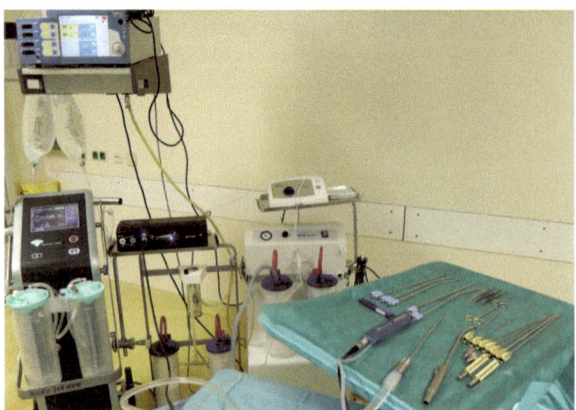

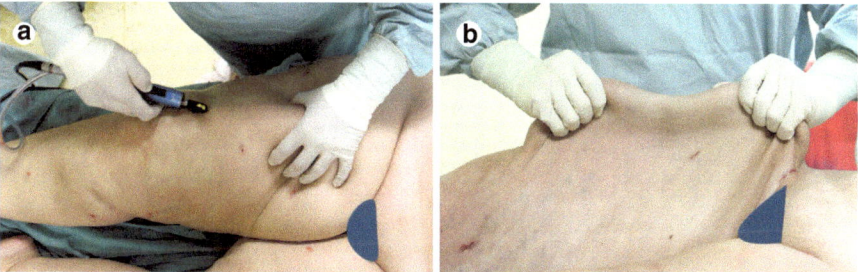

Fig. 3.28 Suctioned thighs during (**a**) and at the end (**b**) of the operation

Fig. 3.29 At the end of
liposuction without
lower leg

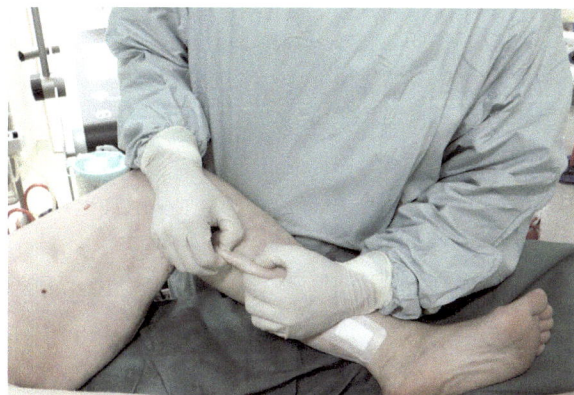

Fig. 3.30 After
liposuction of the arms

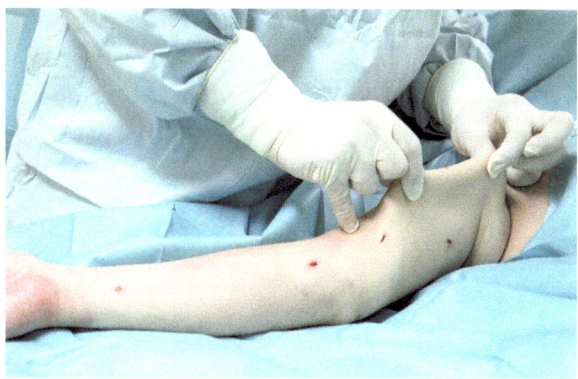

Whether and how many punctures are closed varies from plastic surgeon to plastic surgeon. Some colleagues do not suture the puncture sites at all so that the remains of the saline solution introduced can drain out unhindered. We tend to suture some of the small incisions with dissolving suture material and leave others open. We are moving more and more toward inserting drains. We remove these as soon as the flow rate is less than 30 mL over 24 h. At the end of the operation, sometimes there is taping and application of the compression garment or wrapping for compression treatment. But some form of compression garment should usually be applied to help counteract swelling and bruising. To be fair, there are colleagues who do not use compression and do not have poor results. We always forgo compression when there is a contraindication, a reason why compression should not be applied. Examples are severely wrinkled skin with constrictions or allergic reactions to the material of the compression garment.

On the Day of the Surgery
1. Shower extensively before the operation and put on fresh clothes. This can reduce body contamination with bacteria.
2. Do not apply cream after showering, the marking pen will not hold as well.
3. Refrain from wearing makeup, nail polish, and piercings.
4. Please remove all artificial nails before surgery.
5. In case of surgery on the intimate area, we ask you to shave the area.
6. Do not take sedatives on your own.
7. Discuss in advance which medications you can and cannot take on the day of surgery.
8. Come fasting on the day of surgery (depending on the type of anesthesia).
9. Wear comfortable, loose-fitting clothing on the day of surgery. Make sure that you can easily take off and put on the clothes.

3.7.3　Aftercare

After the operation, you will first be taken to the recovery room to wake up and from there to the ward. If liposuction was planned as an outpatient procedure, you can be driven home after rest and recovery. After surgery, fluid may leak from the small puncture sites. These may also be mixed with blood. The amount of fluid leakage should continuously recede and stop within the first 1–2 days, if not please consult your physician. In the clinic, we keep absorbent pads for you in bed and change them as needed. We also recommend that you use such pads at home. On the Internet, you can find a number of different pads that are suitable for this purpose. Sometimes old towels are absolutely sufficient for this purpose, depending on the volume of fluid leakage.

Painkiller
They are provided with painkillers according to a standard regimen (after querying allergies and intolerances) and receive further adjusted doses of painkillers as needed. Often, NSAIDs, so-called nonsteroidal anti-inflammatory drugs, are sufficient for pain treatment; a well-known active ingredient is ibuprofen. When taking NSAIDs, it is important to have stomach protection, such as omeprazole. For dosage and intake, ask your doctor or pharmacist. Affected persons who have had metabolic surgery are often not allowed to take NSAIDs and must switch to other medications. But let me tell you: Liposuction is usually not very painful.

Fluid Balance

You may get up as soon as you feel like it after liposuction. For the first time, please call a specialist nurse, because there may be circulation problems after liposuction. It is important to drink plenty of fluids after liposuction to help your circulation. This is because the body first fills the suctioned cavities with fluid. In professional circles we call this "volume redistribution." We try to avoid infusions after the procedure as much as possible.

▶ Drink as much as possible in the first days after liposuction.
▶ The shift of fluid into the tissues occurs despite the compression garment, which is designed to counteract swelling.

If you do not drink enough, then water may be removed from the blood, it simply thickens. If the swelling of the leg is added to this, the blood flow back to the heart is inhibited by a squeezing of the blood vessels. In combination with an insufficiently functioning muscle pump of the lower legs due to too little movement (immobilization), the risk of deep vein thrombosis with the danger of developing a pulmonary embolism increases. By drinking and, if necessary, infusions, we can help the fluid balance—the only thing missing is the support of the muscle pump in the lower legs. You can support this with your own exercises by moving your feet to the tip of your nose while lying down and then stretching them.

To counteract thrombosis, you will be given a drug in syringe form for thrombosis prophylaxis. It is usually a low-molecular-weight heparin preparation that is injected once daily. You will receive the first injection on the day of surgery. The injection is given into the subcutaneous fat tissue and into an area that has not been suctioned. In the case of liposuction of the legs, it is recommended to inject into the subcutaneous fatty tissue of the legs and vice versa. We advise performing thrombosis prophylaxis for at least 1 week. Please discuss this with your attending physician. Iron supplements should be continued, if necessary until the iron balance has normalized.

If the legs have been suctioned, it is advisable to keep the legs elevated (e.g., on a pillow) at the beginning consistently and then later in the course in between, so that the swelling and bruising can be transported away to the body more easily. A flexion in the knee joints of more than 80° is counterproductive for the venous return of the blood to the heart. A bend in the knees of about 45° is ideal. This can be achieved well with one or more pillows on the sofa or bed.

▶ Keep elevating the legs/arms every now and then to counteract the swelling.

Lymphatic Drainage

We recommend starting early with lymphatic drainage. Lymphatic drainage is a manual treatment in which excess tissue water is massaged out of the tissue. Usually, lymphatic drainage is offered and performed by physiotherapists, occupational therapists, or lymphatic therapists. This can be started early after 2–3 days. It is important that the lymphatic drainage is painless and that you do not have any circulatory problems. If you feel pain during lymphatic drainage, you should give the internal wounds a few more days to recover and try a new attempt with lymphatic drainage a few days later. One hour of lymphatic drainage costs between 45 and 60 euros, depending on the region. Ideally, lymphatic drainage should be repeated two to three times a week and continued until most of the swelling has subsided. In case of extreme lipedema, it is recommended to start immediately and to perform it every day. In general, lymphatic drainage is not obligatory after liposuction, but the swelling goes down faster with lymphatic drainage.

Bruises

The bruises disappear within 2–3 weeks, although a slight blue tinge may still be visible. This completely recedes in the following 2–3 weeks. The initial hardening of the suctioned areas slowly dissolves and should be completely gone after 4–6 months at the latest. Massaging the bruises 1 to 2 times a day, carefully at first with heparin ointment (60,000 IU ointment), helps the bruises to dissolve quickly, reduces the swelling, and dissolves the scars that form early. In our opinion, the massage is more important than the ointment. To further support the reduction of swelling, we recommend taking bromelain. Bromelain is extracted from pineapple, it has a decongestant and anti-inflammatory effect.

There is controversy about the necessity of antibiotic treatment in terms of prophylaxis, although science considers a single administration to be useful. Depending on the extent of the operation, we continue prophylactic antibiotics for a few days (1–3) in case of extensive liposuction.

Compression Underwear

After the compression garment is applied in the surgery, it should be worn consistently for 23 h a day for at least 8 weeks. Swelling after liposuction increases in the first 2 to 3 days and has its maximum extension about the third day. After that, the swelling process begins, at first quickly, then more and more slowly. Most of the swelling is reduced after 6–8 weeks. Any remaining residual swelling then subsides from the third to the sixth month. If the cost of the surgery is covered by health insurance, you may be given a prescription for a second supply of compression garments. Otherwise, a second suit can be purchased at a medical supply store. A control of the suctioned areas is performed as needed. We check them on the first or second day after the operation, depending on the extent of the liposuction.

▶ The compression garment should be worn for 23 h a day.

The First Shower

A frequent question is: "When can I start showering again?" Here there are quite different statements and opinions in professional circles. We recommend the first shower after 2–3 days, but depending on how you feel, it is also possible earlier. The following things should be taken into account: When you want to take off the compression garment for the first time, for example, for showering, we recommend that you do it in a lying position (bed, sofa, or similar). Beforehand, you should have eaten something light and small and drunk enough throughout the entire period. Furthermore, it is important that a person helps you or is at least in the immediate vicinity, as opening the compression garment can cause circulatory weakness. Likewise, increased fluid may enter the connective tissue of the suctioned areas, resulting in a volume shift in your fluid balance. Dizziness, "black before the eyes" and/or nausea may occur. Therefore, it is good to have someone by your side to help you if needed.

After removing the compression suit, you should first sit carefully on the edge of the bed and wait briefly so that the circulation can adapt to this position. After a few minutes, you then move to a standing position. Before you start walking directly, stand still for a short time and again wait for your body's adaptation reaction. Only start walking when your body gives you the "ok" signal.

Keep showers very short in the first few days and do not shower too hot, as this can also hit the circulation. Showering may be done with shampoo and shower gel before quickly exiting the shower. Dry off and put on a fresh change of clothes. The old suit may be washed in the meantime. We have often heard that some people shower with their suits on, but we do not recommend this. For showering in the first days, shower plasters can be stuck on the wounds. After showering, the shower plasters should be removed.

Follow-Up Checks
After discharge from the hospital, further treatment will take place on an outpatient basis with your plastic surgeon. Depending on the surgery and length of inpatient stay, you should initially see your doctor weekly or as needed. After the third week, we recommend longer intervals between check-ups—every 2–3 weeks if still necessary, then after 8 weeks and after 6–9 months for the final checkup. If you have any problems, questions, or complaints, we recommend seeing your surgeon promptly. You should not carry any worries with you. Your small wounds are usually covered with a band-aid. Change the plasters every 1–2 days at first. Once the wounds are closed, you will not need any more plasters.

Movement
Early mobilization is important to get the circulation going. You should also gradually increase light physical activity. Our motto for this is: move yes, strain no. You should refrain from swimming for at least 4–6 weeks if you have extensive suction. Light sporting activities such as walking are possible after 2–3 weeks. Excessive sports should also wait 4–6 weeks.

Depending on the occupational activity and the amount extracted, work can be resumed after a few days or weeks. In the case of extensive suctioning, you will need at least 3–4 weeks to return to your daily work routine.

Scars

Depending on the surgeon, the small incisions (skin punctures) may or may not have been sutured. If they have been sutured, the suture material may be self-dissolving or non-self-dissolving. If the suture material is non-self-dissolving, the sutures must be removed after 10–12 days. Talk to your doctor about this.

The calling card of a plastic surgeon is the scar that remains in the area of visible skin after each surgical procedure. In liposuction, generally only very small skin incisions are made. However, not all of them are usually closed, which can leave widened scars. Scars can be very different. Ideally, a scar is inconspicuous, flat, pale, fine, soft, and painless. In the opposite case, the scar may be conspicuous, raised, reddened, widened, hardened, and painful. Weather sensitivity is also a typical scar complaint. In addition to uncomplicated scar healing or scar maturation with a desired beautiful scar, we distinguish pathological forms of scars, which are called "hypertrophic" or "keloid" scars.

The following factors can influence scar healing:

– Individual congenital disposition of the scar healing process.
– Localization and positioning of the scar.
– Technique of suturing the wound or leaving it open.
– Tension of the scar during wound closure.
– Suture material.
– Immobilization of the scar for healing.
– Wound care and condition.
– Compression and silicone pads.
– Sun exposure.
– Scar massage.

One of the best and most effective means of scar treatment (by scar is meant the wound suture after the last crust has fallen off) is treatment with silicone and compression. Silicone has been tested in many studies as an effective means of preventing and treating scarring.

The mechanism of action has not yet been conclusively clarified. One important mechanism of action appears to be water vapor transmission (water vapor release). Others suspect a change in the charge in the scar. Normal skin has a transmission of about 8.5 g/m^2 of water vapor per hour. Hypertrophic scars and poorly healing scars have a much lower transmission of about 4.5 g/m^2. The silicone (foil or gel) creates a seal, which positively influences the water vapor emission of the scar. Silicone gel is applied thinly one to two times a day. Silicone foils remain on the scars under compression for at least 6 months to 2 years. The silicone film should be washed off daily with normal hand soap, and the silicone overlay must be boiled for 5 min once a week. Good silicone products have a very long shelf life.

▶ As long as a scar is still reddened and raised, the scar is in the active maturation phase and is organizing itself. In this phase, the scar can still be treated very well with conservative measures such as silicone overlay and compression.

Protect your scar from sun rays. UV rays can cause pigmentation disorders and also hypertrophic scars. Therefore, we recommend avoiding sun radiation or applying sunscreen with at least factor 30 to the scar region. The sunscreen should be applied for at least 1 year.

Active scar massage can prevent unsightly scarring. After initial healing of the scar, daily scar massage can make the scar softer and smoother. Massage improves blood circulation to the scar. This positively affects the fluid metabolism of the scar and the collagen of the scar becomes softer, elastic, and flexible, lowering the initial raised level of the scar.

We recommend you three massage directions: circular, horizontal, and vertical massage. It is possible to use a moisturizing lotion to improve lubrication. Likewise, it is possible to massage the silicone gel while applying it. In doing so, bring two to three fingers together and perform circular movements with light pressure on the scar in the circular massage. In the horizontal method, you massage the scar from one end to the other. In the vertical massage, light up and down movements are used. You should alternate between these different techniques during the massage.

Aftercare after Liposuction

1. At home, use absorbent pads or old towels to soak up any leaking tumescent solution.
2. You will receive an adapted pain therapy.
3. The first time you get up (with the compression on), it is best to do it accompanied as follows: From lying down, you first move to sitting and remain seated at the edge of the bed for a short time. Only when you can cope well with this do you stand up carefully and remain standing in front of the bed for a moment. Then you can take your first steps.
4. Drink enough fluids.
5. Perform daily thromboprophylaxis for at least 1 week.
6. Perform thromboprophylaxis exercises in bed and standing.
7. Continue taking iron supplements after surgery until your blood levels stabilize.
8. If legs or arms have been suctioned, place them high (preferably on pillows) after liposuction.
9. Lymphatic drainage is allowed immediately after surgery but is usually tolerable from the fourth to seventh day. Lymphatic drainage should be painless.
10. Massage bruises with heparin ointment (60,000 IU) daily in the morning and evening, for which they briefly remove the compression garment.
11. We recommend taking decongestant medication, for example, with the active ingredient bromelain.
12. It is usually not necessary to take antibiotics after surgery.

13. Consistently wear your compression garment 23 h a day if possible. In case of constriction or discomfort, it should be taken off. In such a case, consult your doctor. We recommend wearing the garment for at least 8 weeks.
14. A control of the suctioned areas is carried out as required and agreed upon.
15. If you were discharged with a drain, you will need to see your practitioner or physician closely until it is removed.
16. The first time you take off the compression completely (usually after 1–3 days) and then want to stand up, take off the compression while lying down, and then proceed as for the first time standing up.
17. You may shower after the operation. Due to hygienic principles, never shower with the compression on. This must be removed beforehand. Shower for the first time with a companion. We recommend shower plasters at the beginning.
18. Change the plasters every 1–2 days. Once the wounds are closed, you no longer need plasters.
19. Exercise yes, strain no! As soon as it is possible, you should mobilize and move a lot; however, strain should be avoided.
20. In case of severe pain (especially in the calf region), shortness of breath, or shortness of breath, immediately present yourself to us or the attending physician.
21. Use silicone gel for scar treatment and massage your scar.
22. Protect your scars from harmful sunlight with UV protection.

3.7.4   Success and Long-Term Prospects

All sufferers are interested in the lasting effect of liposuction. But is liposuction for lipedema really sustainable? There is no general answer to this question. As almost always, it depends on the initial situation. If there is pronounced obesity at the beginning of treatment, which is not treated, and there is no treatment plan for obesity, then liposuction is unlikely to be crowned with long-term success. It is exactly these patients who report in the aftermath that immediately after the surgery it starts to "proliferate" on the abdomen or in other regions. However, it does not proliferate, the excess calories are deposited differently than before the operation due to the changed fat cell count and fat precursor cell count and their distribution.

In cases of only mild obesity involving fat distribution disorder and nonobese sufferers, a simple lifestyle and dietary change combined with liposuction as defined by our complex surgical treatment may be the key to long-term success.

There is almost always a significant improvement or even a complete decrease in pain after treatment. However, depending on whom you ask, different opinions prevail about the effectiveness of liposuction, especially in the long-term course. Freedom from complaints after liposuction is stated quite differently in various studies from 100 to 70 to 20%. No study stands out qualitatively enough to say that this is the study that can be trusted.

From our point of view, liposuction for lipedema or even for the existence of pure lipohypertrophy has a really very good prognosis to be long-term and sustainable. With successful treatment, one certainly improves first of all the physical complaints including the mobility and the ability to bear weight, but there is also a significant improvement of the body shape. The improved body shape almost always leads to mental stabilization, an increase in self-confidence, and more participation in social and working life. To answer the question of sustainability: the indication and the therapy plan must be right.

▶ When properly indicated, the results of liposuction are usually long-term and sustainable.

If there is a complete reduction in the symptoms of lipedema as a result of weight loss, conservative therapy or complex surgical treatment alone, many people speak of lipedema in remission. Remission because those affected continue to carry the predisposition to lipedema. It can therefore never be ruled out that removed fatty tissue will come back in the same place and lead to renewed lipedema symptoms. No one can guarantee success.

More often than a recurrence or worsening of lipedema, we are told by affected women that they could really lose weight for the first time after liposuction. We do not know in detail what is responsible for this, but certainly, the breaking of the hormonal regulatory circuit of the adipose tissue plays a major role. Likewise, intrinsic, newfound motivation certainly plays an important role. Liposuction removes not rigid but hormone-active adipose tissue.

The success of liposuction varies depending on the region. We have some regions that we refer to internally as "problem regions " and "difficult to suction." The front of the knee (Fig. 3.31) and lower leg are particularly worthy of mention here.

The problem with knee joints is that the excess fat in this region is highly septated. These septa make liposuction enormously difficult. Furthermore, there is often connective tissue fibrosis in this area. However, there are two additional factors: (1) the skin recedes more poorly in this area than in other regions and (2.) the remaining excess skin overlaps the knee joint due to the firm connective tissue fibers around the knee joint.

Another "problem region" is the front and back of the lower leg. Due to the frequently advanced fibrosis here as well, the tissue cannot always be removed as desired and residual tissue swelling remains (Fig. 3.32).

The last problem region is the waist–abdomen–hip transition. In particular, if only the hips and extremities are suctioned without shaping the waist and abdominal region, a harmonious transition is often not possible. However, this is purely an aesthetic aspect.

Often women affected by lipedema also suffer from cellulite (please do not confuse it with cellulitis! Cellulitis, in contrast to cellulite, is a bacterial inflammation of the subcutaneous connective tissue). Cellulite is caused by the female sex hormone estrogen and appears as so-called orange peel skin with dents and waves, especially on the buttocks and hips. Cellulite in itself is not a disease and does not cause pain on its own.

Fig. 3.31 Problem zone
knee joint region

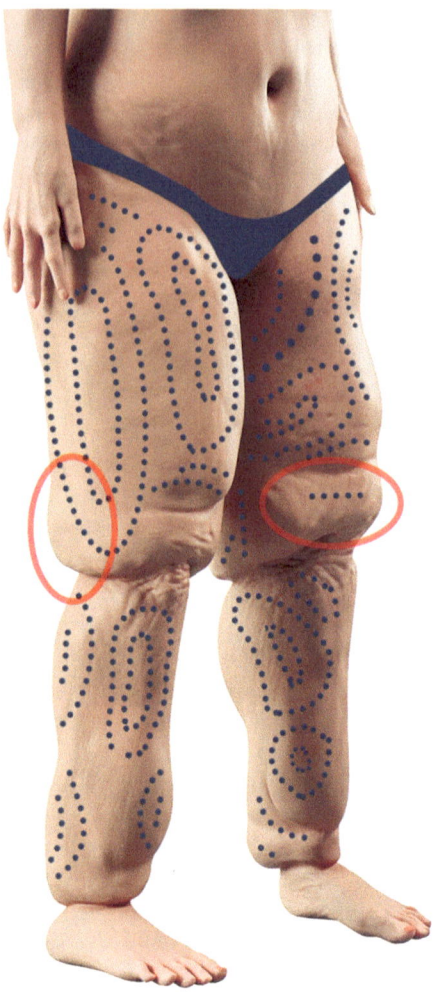

As we read in Sect. 1.2.1, the subcutaneous fat tissue is separated from each other by connective tissue fibers (septa). In contrast to men, the septa are arranged differently in women. In women, the rather fine connective tissue septa run perpendicular to the skin surface, whereas in men they run parallel and crosswise. This makes men's skin more robust and stable, while women's skin is softer and more flexible, which is advantageous during pregnancy, for example. Overall, however, this makes women's skin less resistant to the underlying fatty tissue.

As a result, the fatty tissue can push up to the upper layers of the skin and cause bulging. Liposuction results in several effects on cellulite, which can be treated positively in the long term. The causing fat pads are removed and the connective tissue fibers are slightly injured. This leads to scarring and stabilization of the fat pads. These two effects lead to a regular improvement of the skin appearance after liposuction (Fig. 3.33). We do not show before and after pictures due to the law on

Fig. 3.32 Problem zone lower leg

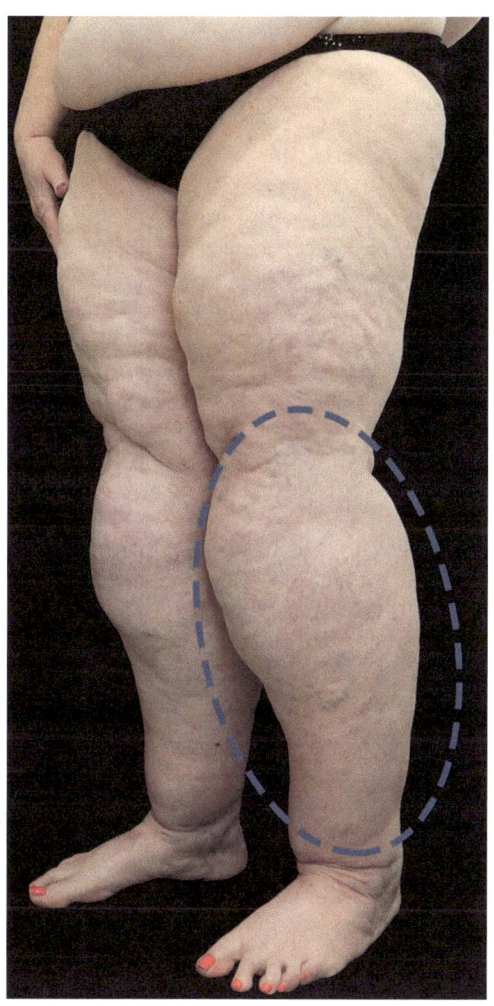

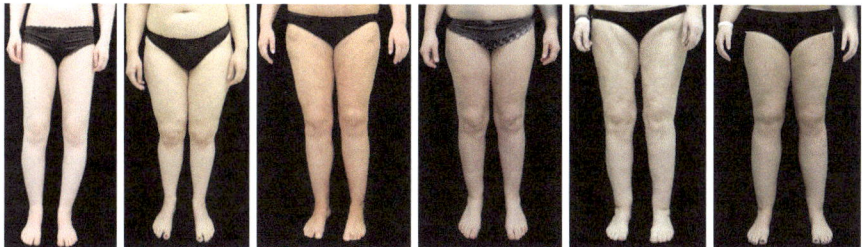

Fig. 3.33 Results of liposuction for lipedema

advertising of medical products. However, these can be shown to you during a personal consultation with your doctor.

3.7.5   Consequences and Risks

We have already talked about the positive aspects of liposuction. But what about the consequences and risks? Depending on how much fatty tissue is suctioned out, there is a risk of tissue slackening, that is, sagging of the skin. This is where our skin plays a central role. The skin is our largest human, organ and, in addition to its barrier function against environmental influences, has many other functions, such as temperature and water balance regulation. The skin consists of different layers, roughly subdivided, the epidermis and the dermis or corium (Fig. 3.34).

Simplified, the structure of the skin (Fig. 3.34) can be imagined as many individual skin cells, which individually look like a brick, lying next to and on top of each other like a brick facade. The cells grow from the depths toward the surface, undergo a maturation process, and are shed on the surface as skin scales.

The basis of skin elasticity is collagen fibers and elastin. These are also known as fibrous protein and are located in the dermis (deep layer of skin), run parallel to the surface of the body, and together form a matrix (network compound). The combination of elastin and collagen results in the elasticity and tear resistance of the tissue. However, this elasticity and tensile strength are finite and therefore limited. If this matrix is overstretched and destroyed, the stretch marks we are all familiar with will appear. In technical jargon, these are also called "striae distensae." Externally, these areas of overstretching appear as blue-reddish stripes. The coloration is the result of an on-site inflammatory reaction caused by the tearing. The skin at the tearing site becomes thinner than in other areas so that the small skin vessels show through and are responsible for a change in color in this region. To some extent, these streaks fade over time, but the overused skin has lost the ability to regress. After illustrating

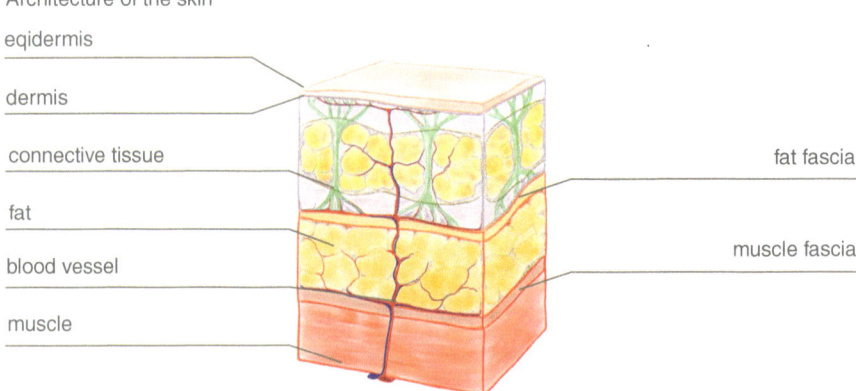

Fig. 3.34 Structure of the skin

this mechanism of tearing, it also becomes understandable that a cream or lotion cannot really help repair the complex.

If volume removal occurs in the subcutaneous fat tissue, the outer mantle (the skin) must adapt to the new volume. The extent to which your skin recedes is very individual. Here, the inherited skin quality with its regression property certainly plays a very central role. Surprisingly, in some patients, the skin recedes massively and very well (in Fig. 3.35, we show a good skin shrinkage result after liposuction of many liters on the legs), in others even a small loss of volume is sufficient for the formation of sagging skin.

You may wonder whether there are any measures that can positively influence the desired skin shrinkage process through external factors. Exercise and nutrition play a central role here. Exercise promotes tissue circulation and supports the natural metabolic balance in the long term. Likewise, a balanced diet rich in vitamins is an essential basic building block for the regeneration of skin and tissue.

Fig. 3.35 Result after liposuction

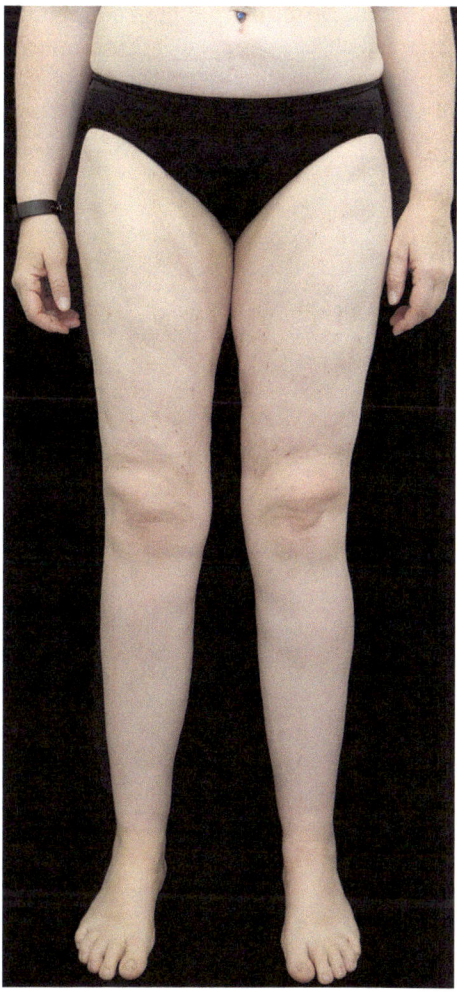

You should avoid smoking at all costs. Smoking causes the skin to age faster and reduces the skin's metabolism. Likewise, excessive sun exposure is harmful to your skin. Massaging the skin with oils and creams rich in vitamins (e.g., vitamins A, B3, C, E, and H) is quite useful. However, we see the positive effect more in the local massage and increase in tissue circulation than through the active ingredients per se.

What can we say in conclusion about the probability of skin shrinkage after liposuction for lipedema? Depending on the type of skin and the region suctioned, the skin behaves differently and therefore recedes differently well, but it is not possible to predict with certainty what it will actually be like against the background of the above-mentioned reasons.

▶ The elasticity of the skin is finite. After reaching the elasticity limit, stretch marks, wrinkles, and sagging skin develop. Each region of the body reacts differently.

In general, the inner thighs quickly begin to sag. In contrast, the outer sides of the hips and upper arms compensate for sagging quite well, up to a certain extent.

It is not always easy to strike a balance between residual fat, hanging skin, and aesthetics, although in lipedema we recommend and usually perform maximum fat reduction because of the existing pain (Fig. 3.36).

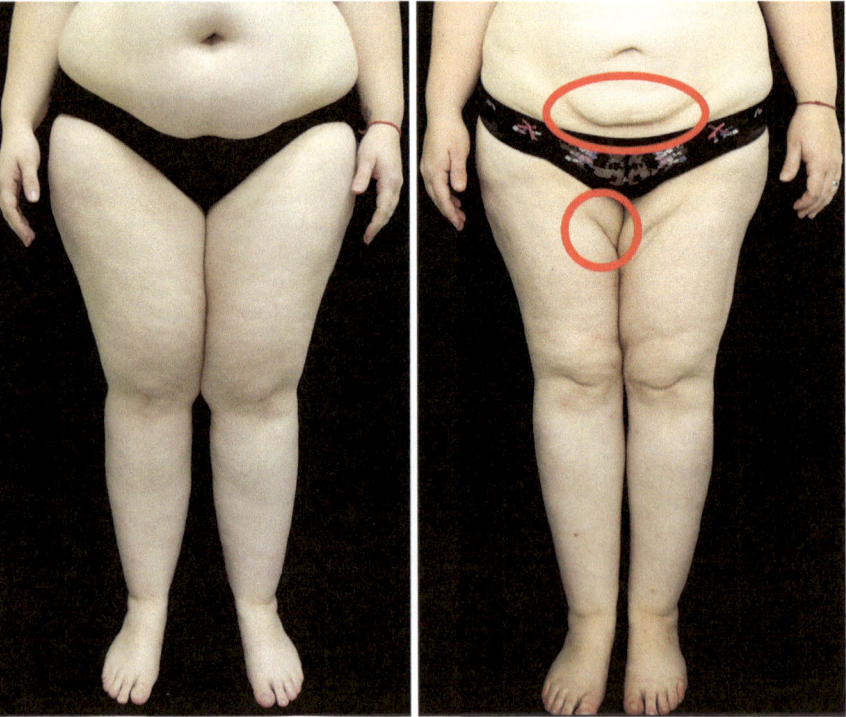

Fig. 3.36 Sagging skin on abdomen and legs after liposuction of 30 L of pure adipose tissue on legs, abdomen, arms, and back over three sessions

Why are we even talking about the issue of sagging skin? Sagging and wrinkled skin can also cause problems. Skin irritation and restricted movement are the most frequently expressed and seen complaints. Areas of skin that lie on top of each other cause heat to build up and, in the absence of air circulation, a moist chamber is formed, disrupting the natural skin barrier. In the worst case, redness or sores can be the result.

Excess "skin flaps," especially on the upper arms and thighs, can restrict natural movement in everyday life and especially during sports. The excess lags behind the arm and leg movement due to its inherent inertia.

None of those affected likes to undress in front of others and "present" their excess skin. This results in the exclusion of many activities, for example, swimming, sunbathing on the beach, or even just wearing short fashionable clothes. Likewise, in many sufferers, the partnership suffers and not in a small way. We speak of social isolation, psychological stress, and withdrawal from the social environment with isolation.

Important: You should talk about possible tissue sagging after surgery with your doctor before liposuction. Most plastic surgeons address this topic on their own initiative, while other groups of doctors, who do not perform lifting operations themselves, sometimes like to leave this topic out. Don't be fobbed off with phrases like "it almost never happens" or "we'll talk about it then."

In patients who are fairly certain to experience skin sagging, we already include these tightening operations in our initial therapy plan to create transparency. Overall, although we perform tightening surgeries very frequently, they are rather rare in lipedema patients compared to patients after massive weight loss due to gastric surgery. We include the group of extremely obese lipedema patients in the group of patients after massive weight loss. Even if lipedema is still worth treating after weight loss, skin slackening due to the mass is still in the foreground.

Let's move on to the risks. Every surgeon who operates also has complications. If he doesn't have any, he doesn't operate or he fibs. Good complication management is an important quality feature of a good specialist.

The so-called clarification meeting must take place at least 24 hours before the operation. Even if you have signed this clarification, you can withdraw from the operation at any time without stating a reason. As a rule, you must not incur any costs by canceling the operation, regardless of whether the costs of the operation are borne by the health insurance company or by yourself.

The risks listed here are only an excerpt of possible surgical risks. Your attending physician must discuss any special risks you may have in detail with you before the operation.

First of all, we will go into very general risks. Every operation that involves anesthesia is associated with an anesthetic risk. This will be explained to you in detail by the anesthesiologist during the anesthesia consultation.

General surgical risks are as follows: Despite the greatest care, blood vessels can be injured during liposuction. Some injuries can never be avoided, but they should be as minimal as possible. After the procedure, there is always further fluid leakage through the puncture sites. Often the fluid is diluted with blood. If there is more bleeding after the operation, they form larger and extensive bruises. As described in Section 0, postoperative bleeding and/or thinning of the blood may necessitate a blood transfusion. In our case, it happens about once per year that a blood transfusion is necessary, despite very high to extremely high lipoaspirate volumes.

A distinction must be made between how extensive and how voluminous liposuction is performed. Let us consider the following actual scenario with two different liposuction procedures: Patient 1, normal weight with very mild visually pronounced lipedema but severe pain, Patient 2 with extreme lipedema, mild obesity, and moderate pain. Patient 1 receives liposuction on her arms, legs, front and back, that is, very extensive liposuction with a suction volume of 3.5 L of pure fatty tissue. Patient 2 receives liposuction only on the front of the legs (11.8 L of pure adipose tissue). Of course, the second patient has significantly more fat deposits than the other, and one would theoretically have to list further details such as body size, general condition, and many more, at this point, but we will refrain from doing so here. In short, patient 1 (3.5 L) experienced greater blood loss due to areal hemorrhage combined with greater dilution. The consequences were dizziness, ringing in the ears, headache, nausea, palpitations, and general weakness. Hb was 6 mg/dl and hematocrit was 20%. A blood transfusion was necessary. The subject was quite weak on her feet for 1 week; the other got up on the day of surgery, had a perfect course, and went home 2 days later. This means that it often depends on the extent of liposuction and not on the amount.

▶   The volume aspirated alone does not reflect the risk.

Despite high-quality controls of blood products, a blood transfusion is associated with the risk, albeit very low, of transmission of infectious diseases. Other risks of blood transfusion include allergic shock reactions, chills, headaches, muscle cramps, fever, and fatigue. Autologous blood donation and subsequent administration of autologous blood are no longer performed. We consider the risk of blood transfusion during liposuction to be very low.

In addition to extensive hemorrhage, we distinguish acute local hemorrhage. This can happen when a larger blood vessel is injured. In my entire career, I have experienced this one time. In the affected person, liposuction for the planned upper arm lift was performed in one session. Through the tube, we could see a clear unusual blood leakage and then found an injured blood vessel through the incision of the upper arm lift. Even if no lift had been planned, we would have had to make an incision to stop the bleeding.

Bruising occurs in most liposuction procedures, that is a fact. Other risks are dents and waves in the sense of irregularities of the suctioned areas. These may also require correction if severe. The risk of dents and ripples is greater in very voluminous liposuction procedures than in others.

Liposuction can theoretically injure lymphatic vessels, especially if sharp cannulas are used. I personally have not seen any liposuction-induced lymphedema— neither in our lymphedema consultation nor in our lipedema consultation.

Occasionally, there is circumscribed loss of sensation due to injury to small cutaneous nerves. These sensory losses usually regenerate slowly over 2 years.

Extremely rarely do we see infections or healing disorders of the wound and even more rarely they spread. In the worst case, these could develop into blood poisoning. This would be a serious complication requiring inpatient or even intensive care treatment.

Circumscribed or local wound healing disorders are usually treated conservatively, that is, without surgery. Treatment includes regular wound cleansing, application of disinfecting ointment, and application of clean dressings. An example of disinfecting ointment is Lavanid gel. However, the "brand" is not decisive, but the ingredient should be polyhexanide 0.04% or 0.02%. In case of infection or wound healing disorder, an antibiotic in tablet form may be recommended. You should follow this recommendation without fail.

▶ If there is a wound-healing problem, see your plastic surgeon and discuss wound treatment.

A complication that we see more frequently with very extensive liposuction and almost exclusively in the area of the outer thighs isaccumulation of wound water, so-called seromas. Often the problem resolves itself, but sometimes we have to puncture the seromas in the consultation. Occasionally we insert drains. Up to now, we have always managed to get all seromas under control. To be able to answer the legitimate question as to why the seromas only occur on the outer sides of the thighs, we must first look at Fig. 3.37. Here you can see that exactly in the outer thigh region there are no lymphatic channels and therefore no lymphatic collectors. Therefore, tissue water that accumulates there can be poorly removed. An accumulation of tissue water (seroma) can therefore develop preferentially in this region.

With every operation, there is a risk of suffering a thrombosis or pulmonary embolism during or after the operation. In thrombosis, the blood thickens after surgery due to the loss of blood or fluid. This causes local swelling that squeezes blood vessels and reduces blood flow back to the heart. Blood vessel injury and activation of the body's clotting system also play a role in the development of thrombosis. In addition, being bedridden causes the circulatory system to shut down. This and other reasons are responsible for the development of thrombosis. If thrombosis occurs, it is usually in the veins of the lower leg. From there, a thrombus can detach from the vessel and travel via the heart to the lungs. The migration of the thrombus to the lungs occurs via the pulmonary artery, hence the name "pulmonary artery embolism." Once in the lung, the thrombus—depending on whether it blocks a large or small vessel—cuts off that area of the lung from its function of supplying the blood with oxygen. A pulmonary embolism is an emergency that requires intensive medical care and, in the worst case, can result in death. To prevent thrombosis, you should drink enough to counteract blood thickening.

Another important goal is to improve venous return to the heart. This is possible via the following physical measures:

– Compression suit/compression stockings.
– Wrap dressing.
– Pneumatic leg cuffs.

Fig. 3.37 Seromes

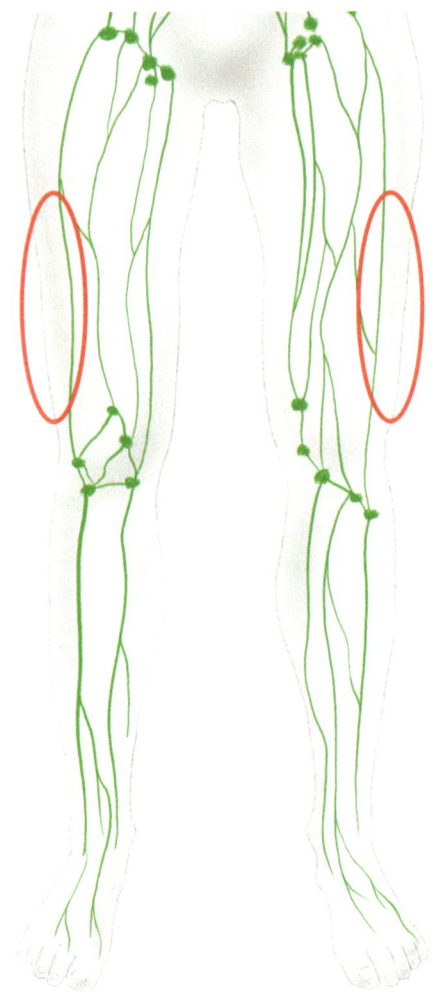

– Legs up.
– Early mobilization.
– Exercise therapy, such as bed exercises.

You will be put on the compression suit after the surgery in the operating room, sometimes with an additional wrapping bandage. In bed, your legs should be elevated. After the operation, it is important that you mobilize as soon as possible. As soon as you can sit at the edge of the bed without any problems, they should move to standing as early as possible, first under escort and then alone. Stop short of the bed and listen to your body. It will tell you if you can already take your first steps, first at room level and then at ward level. Walking is of immense importance, as it

Fig. 3.38 Exercise for
thrombosis prophylaxis

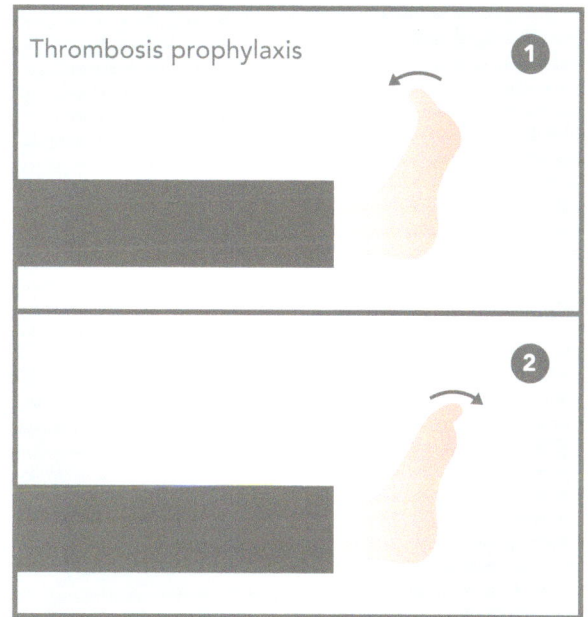

not only stimulates circulation but also activates the muscle pump in the calves. The muscle pump in the calves supports a return flow of blood from the legs to the heart.

But also movement exercises in bed help to prevent thrombosis. For this purpose, we would like to give you two exercises that you can do alone in bed.

Exercise number 1 (Fig. 3.38): You lie relaxed in bed with your arms placed loosely beside your body. Your legs are stretched out in bed and the tips of your toes point upwards. Now bend and stretch your toes as shown in Fig. 3.38 15 times.

Exercise number 2 (Fig. 3.39): As soon as you can sit, sit on a chair and place your feet on the floor. Press the heels of both feet firmly on the floor and lift the tops of the feet vigorously. Keep the tips of your toes up briefly. Then roll over the tips of your toes with pressure. Repeat this exercise 15 times as well. Try to do the exercises several times a day.

Summary thrombosis prophylaxis
- Take in sufficient fluids (drinking, infusions).
- Movement and exercises for the muscles of the lower legs.
- Prophylaxis injection for at least 4 days.
- Compression garments.

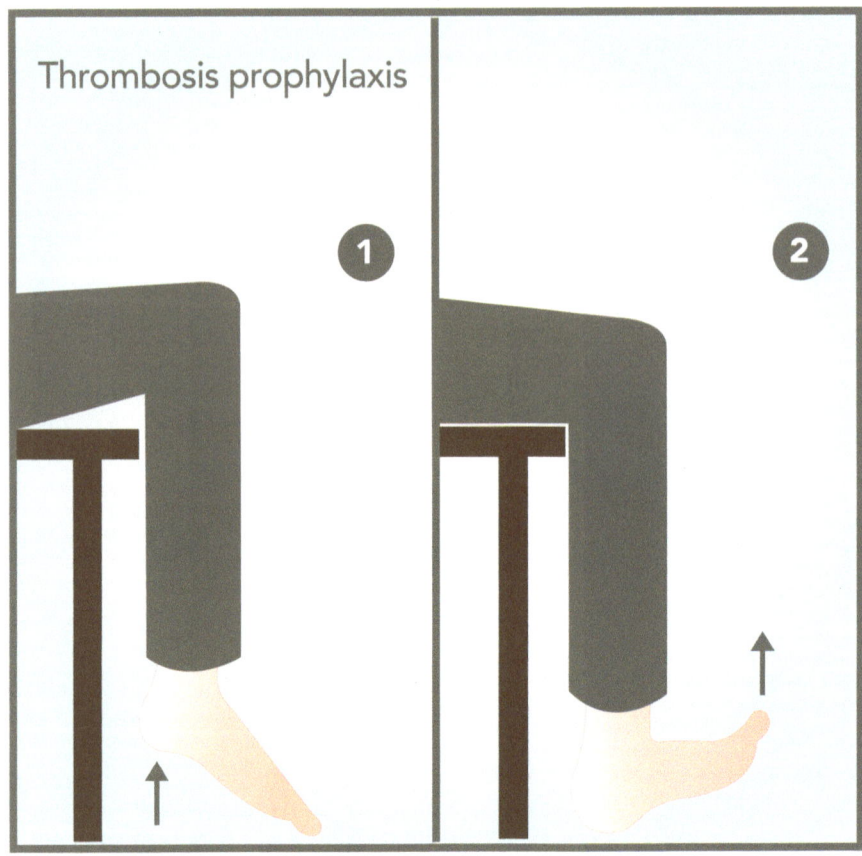

Fig. 3.39 Exercise for thrombosis prophylaxis

Symptoms of Possible Thrombosis
- Increasing swelling of the legs with a feeling of heaviness and/or tension.
- Pain in the leg, often especially in the lower legs in the area of the calves (pressure pain).
- Overheating or blue discoloration of the skin.

▶ If you have symptoms that make you suspect you may have a thrombosis, please present to your doctor or an emergency room immediately.

A thrombosis can develop into a pulmonary embolism with far-reaching consequences, such as intensive medical treatment or, in the worst case, death. A patient dying during liposuction is an extremely rare complication, and we don't want to scare you. However, the rare complications must also be addressed, because no one can rule out a complication in advance.

"Take a deep breath" is the motto. After a procedure, pain can be responsible for your inability to breathe properly. This can lead to lung ventilation problems or, even worse, pneumonia. But not only deep breathing, but also exercises with the so-called Triflow help to ventilate the lungs well.

▶   Ask the hospital for a Triflow to do your breathing exercises.

To perform the lung ventilation exercise with the Triflow, place the mouthpiece of the Triflow in your mouth (Fig. 3.40), seal the mouthpiece with your lips and inhale so deeply that the balls slowly rise up one after the other (Fig. 3.41). It is better to hold only one or two balls up for as long as possible than to hastily try to pull all three balls up. It is best to repeat this exercise every hour, trying to pull the balls up more than 5 times. Rotate the Triflow and exhale. Likewise, try to keep all the balls up as long as possible.

▶   If you have trouble breathing or any of the symptoms listed in the overview, please present to your doctor or an emergency room immediately.

This was an excerpt of possible complications and risks. Before surgery, a detailed discussion will take place in which you will be informed about these and other risks.

Fig. 3.40 Triflow exercise: Inserting the mouthpiece

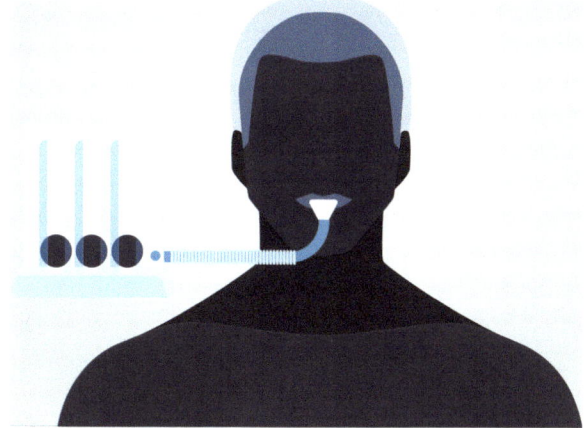

Fig. 3.41 Triflow
exercise: take a deep breath

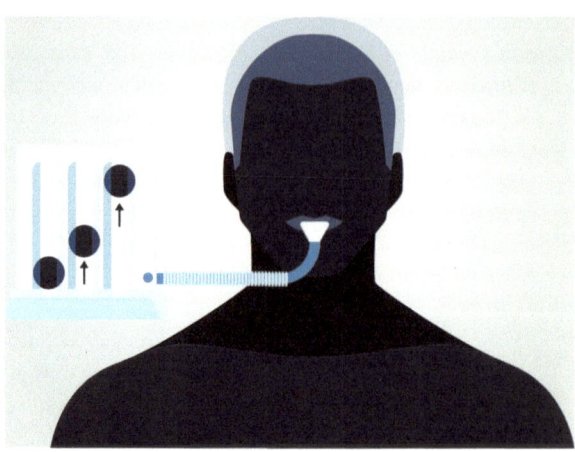

Possible Symptoms of Pulmonary Artery Embolism

– Shortness of breath when inhaling or exhaling, possibly accelerated
  breathing.
– Pain when breathing and chest pain, which may also radiate.
– Palpitations.
– Anxiety, possibly with sweating.
– Dizziness, fatigue, fainting.
– Cough and/or hemoptysis.
– Unusual sounds when breathing.

3.7.6 Course of the Complex-Operative Therapy Plan

Many people wonder in which order the liposuctions is performed. Let us now go into the sequence of the complex surgical therapy plan and especially the sequence of the planned liposuctions integrated into it.

The complex-surgical treatment plan includes:

1. Conservative treatment of lipedema with compression therapy, if necessary lymphatic drainage, if edema should be present (optional).
2. Weight analysis and, if necessary, treatment of concomitant obesity (from lifestyle modification to metabolic surgery).
3. Liposuctions for the treatment of lipedema.
4. Tightening surgery for foreseeable, physically limiting skin-soft tissue excess.

In the following, we will discuss point 3, how the individual liposuctions proceed.

Many providers of liposuction for lipedema have their own concept of how and in what sequence liposuction is performed. We have our own names for the different procedures: the "bottom-up concept," the "outside-in concept," the "holistic suction concept," the "lipedema compression concept" and the concept of SRL liposuction, systematic-regional liposuction.

"Bottom-up" Concept
In the "bottom-up"concept, the lower parts of the body are suctioned first and the upper part of the body in subsequent operations. An example would be suctioning the lower legs and knee region in one operation; the thighs would be suctioned in a second and finally the hips in a third.

"From the outside in" Concept
In the "from the outside to the inside" concept, liposuction of the outer sides is performed in a first operation and liposuction of the inner sides in another operation. An example here would be liposuction of the lower legs, knees, thighs, and outer sides of the hips first. In the follow-up surgery, the inner sides of the lower leg, knee, and thigh would be suctioned.

"Concept of Holistic Suction".
The "concept of holistic liposuction" suctions all body areas, as the theory is that lipedema "migrates" after liposuction and then affects other areas.

"Lipedema Compression Concept"
The "lipedema compression concept" is interpreted differently. Many suction all areas "somewhat" and again and again in different interventions until a satisfactory result is achieved.

"SRL Liposuction Concept".
SRL stands for "systematic regional liposuction." This concept has emerged after many years of searching for the best approach for us and many plastic surgery colleagues. It includes, among other things, the systematic working off of the affected regions, the sequence of procedures, and the technique of how liposuction is to be performed. It does not matter whether we perform WAL, PAL, or other liposuction.

▶ SRL stands for "systematic-regional liposuction" in which we try to close regions if possible and not suction them twice.

To understand our concept, it is necessary to consider many individual factors. It is necessary to consider how the anatomy is, how liposuction works and is performed, what happens in the body as a result of liposuction and what the healing process is like. Our concept of systematic regional liposuction (SRL liposuction), due to the reasons listed above, always tries to close off regions as much as possible to avoid second and third liposuction of a region. At the same time, we must not disregard aesthetics and must continuously suction the transitions as well. This does not mean that small corrections here and there or even second aspirations cannot occur, but we try to completely aspirate and close a region in one procedure if possible.

But now it still depends on the fat deposits present. If these exceed an appropriate volume, secondary liposuction must be performed in any case. However, in about 70% of cases, we can avoid this.

If we look at a classic case and see that lipedema is significantly located in the hip–thigh region and lower legs, often with a moderate expression, we can reach all affected areas in two liposuctions. One liposuction would then be performed in the supine position and another in the prone position.

▶ Supine position means that you lie on your back during the operation. In the prone position, it is the other way around accordingly.

During these individual liposuctions, we suction off a maximum amount of fatty tissue according to medically justifiable criteria. Of course, transitional areas are always suctioned as well, to obtain a harmonious transition between the regions as far as possible. It is not possible to suction off the entire fatty tissue, that is, completely, without leaving any fatty tissue behind. Those colleagues who advertise or even make these statements must be questioned very critically. However, as little as possible fatty tissue should remain.

▶ A statement like "we can remove all the fatty tissue or all the diseased fatty tissue" is not serious. Give a wide berth to such users.

In the first operation in the supine position, we finally get good access to the outer sides of the hips, the thighs (front, outer, and inner sides) and also the inner sides of the knees. If there is also lipedema on the lower legs, we can treat the front, outer and inner sides of the lower legs as well. This is done until we reach our reasonable volume limits or the maximum duration of surgery (for volume limits Section 0).

The second operation is liposuction in the prone position. In this session, the outer sides of the hips (buttocks if necessary) are again treated and completed as a transitional region. The same applies to the inner thighs. Suction is applied to the backs of the thighs and the transitional region of the inner sides of the knees and the inner and outer sides of the lower legs. We often pay special attention to the lower leg region in this operation. This region, which is the most challenging to suction, requires highly precise work and a lot of experience.

Depending on the extent of the first liposuction, the second liposuction can follow at the earliest after 2 months, better after 3–6 months. A too short interval between liposuctions is not recommended for medium to pronounced liposuctions, since the physical strain is quite high and the bruises and scarring need time to recede. Likewise, personal–social aspects such as career and family should also be taken into account.

If the affected person also suffers from lipedema in the arms, the arms could be combined with liposuction of the backs, but only if it fits from the circumference. Otherwise, the arms would have to be liposuctioned in a separate procedure.

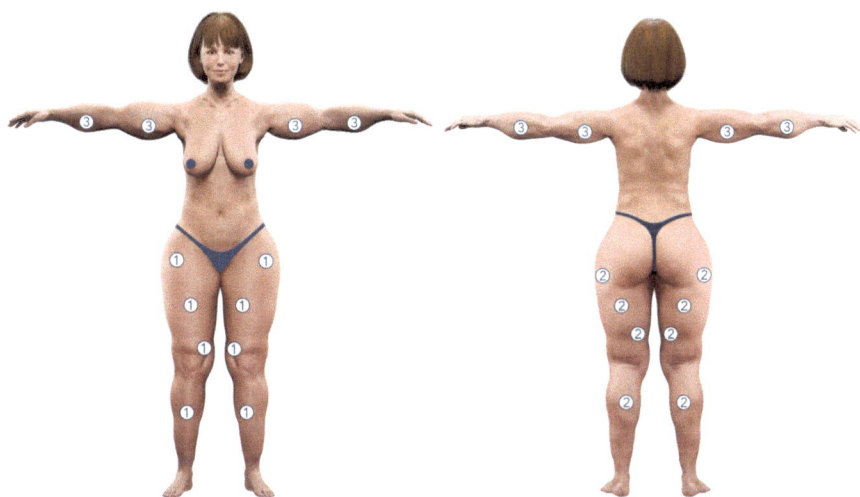

Fig. 3.42 Flowchart of liposuction

A three-stage treatment plan is shown in Fig. 3.42. In the first step, liposuction of the fronts is performed, in the second step, liposuction of the backs is performed, and in the third step, liposuction of the arms is performed.

We recommend an interval of at least 2–3 months between two operations involving the same transition areas. If liposuction of an area is planned more than once due to a strong manifestation of lipedema, we recommend an interval of at least 6 months between the operations.

Some colleagues recommend whole-body liposuction to treat lipedema, that is, liposuction of all areas of the body, because otherwise, lipedema will spread elsewhere on the body. On the one hand, it is nonsensical to argue this way; on the other hand, the approach makes perfect sense, and always when liposuction is used as the sole surgical component. Especially in the case of obese people, the approach is understandable, but it does not promise long-lasting success.

We also very often advise liposuction of more regions than just the arms, buttocks, hips, and legs. However, the overall treatment plan must be correct, and the recommendation of extensive liposuction is purely for aesthetic reasons, and we stand by that. Through extensive liposuction, including the back area, flanks, abdomen, and lateral thoracic wall, we can shape an aesthetic and sophisticated body contour beyond the goal of pure pain treatment.

▶   We often recommend suctioning other areas of the body for purely aesthetic reasons.

In Table 3.5 you will find a few examples of typical liposuction plans to help you understand our planning. Although the treatment plan is fixed, it is flexible in the course and can be readjusted after each procedure. Sometimes this reduces the

Table 3.5 Typical liposuction plans

Stage	Location	Quantity	Extraction area
Lipedema type 4 stage I (hips, legs, and arms)	Supine position	1	Hips
			Outer, anterior, and inner thighs
			Front and inner sides of the knee
			Lower leg front, outer, and inner sides
	Prone position	1	Hips
			Outer, back, and inner thighs
			Inside knee
			Back, outer, and inner sides of the lower leg
			Poor
Lipedema type 3 stage II (hips and legs)	Supine position	1	Hips
			Outer, anterior, and inner thighs
			Front and inner sides of the knee
			Lower leg front, outer, and inner sides
	Prone position	1	Hips
			Outer, back, and inner thighs
			Inside knee
			Back, outer, and inner sides of the lower leg
Lipedema type 3 stage III	Supine position	2 or more	Hips
			Outer, anterior, and inner thighs
			Front and inner sides of the knee
			Lower leg front, outer, and inner sides
			The regions can be further subdivided per OP.
	Prone position	2 or more	Hips
			Outer, back, and inner thighs
			Inside knee
			Back, outer, and inner sides of the lower leg
			The regions can be further divided per surgery. We would alternate between front and then back suction every 2–3 months.
Lipedema type III stage II plus abdominal region, flanks, and back	Supine position	1–2	Hips
			Outer, anterior and inner thighs
			Front and inner sides of the knee
			Lower leg front, outer and inner sides
			The regions can be further subdivided per OP.
	Prone position	1–2	Hips
			Outer, back, and inner thighs
			Inside knee
			Back, outer and inner sides of the lower leg
			Plus liposuction of buttocks, back, and flanks if necessary.
			The regions can be further subdivided per OP.
	Supine position	1	Belly
			Flanks

Table 3.5 (continued)

Stage	Location	Quantity	Extraction area
Lipedema type IV stage II plus abdominal region, flanks, and back	Supine position	1–2	Hips
			Outer, anterior, and inner thighs
			Front and inner sides of the knee
			Lower leg front, outer, and inner sides
			The regions can be further subdivided per OP.
	Prone position	1–2	Hips
			Outer, back, and inner thighs
			Inside knee
			Back, outer, and inner sides of the lower leg
			Plus liposuction of buttocks, back, and flanks if necessary.
			The regions can be further subdivided per OP.
	Supine position	1	Belly
			Flanks
	Supine position	1	Arms (with liposuction on the abdomen and flanks, if necessary).

number of liposuctions planned as the procedure progresses. Any necessary tightening operations are performed after 6 months.

A very frequently asked question is when is the best time for surgerywhen planning to have children. There are different opinions on this and we do not have a general answer. The fear of further aggravation of lipedema is justified and is frequently observed. However, we have also observed worsening of lipedema after liposuction and subsequent pregnancy.

We hold the following opinion: A desire to have children always comes first. For those who do not want to have children for fear of aggravation, we would like to point out that this fear is unjustified, as much can be corrected and achieved afterwards.

It is, therefore, necessary to consider performing liposuction before pregnancy or afterwards. The aim of liposuction before pregnancy would be to remove as much fatty tissue as possible so that there is no significant increase in volume during pregnancy. Liposuction after pregnancy would have the advantage of removing areas that may have worsened.

Following thoughts:

- Not every pregnancy is associated with an exacerbation (probability is high, however).
- Despite liposuction in advance, there may be a significant increase in lipedema.
- Pregnancy often leads to significant tissue sagging, whether with or without liposuction beforehand.
- Much more important than liposuction in advance is a perfect diet and lifestyle during pregnancy. There are special courses and concepts for this.
- After the completion of the childbearing process, a holistic approach to body shape correction, including lipedema treatment, can be created if needed.

My personal opinion: If pregnancy is planned within the next 1–3 years, I would rather not recommend liposuction in advance. If the time is unknown or in the distant future, we recommend lipedema treatment in advance. Finally, it is also a question of cost coverage and financial means.

Conclusion on Surgical Liposuction Treatment for Lipedema Neither conservative nor surgical treatment can cure lipedema. We do not share the classic recommendation that conservative therapy should be exhausted and now consider surgical therapy to be the treatment of choice for the treatment of lipedema, but only with the inclusion of possible obesity in the sense of complex surgical treatment with an individual therapy plan. Likewise, the complex surgical treatment also includes a forward-looking assessment of the impending change in body shape and requires mandatory consideration of possible tightening operations.

3.8   Treatment Example

In the following, we would like to tell you a very classic lipedema patient story: The 36-year-old patient presented for the first time in our outpatient consultation. She reported suffering from a disproportion in favor of the legs and arms since puberty— initially very discreet and only noticeable to herself, but then increasingly. The first attempts at dieting failed, and there was a slow weight gain, almost always after dieting. In addition to the disproportion described, the affected person reported that she experienced pain under stress and later also at rest. At the slightest bump, she suffered a bruise. The disproportion became more pronounced over time. Likewise, the pain worsened. All further attempts to maintain and control the body weight failed. On the contrary, there was a creeping weight gain. The pregnancy of the first and the second child led to a significant aggravation. Especially the pain would have been almost unbearable by now. Many visits to the doctor followed, all of which were disappointing and unsuccessful. Finally, she presented to a vascular surgeon colleague in private practice. The diagnosis was made: lipedema.

Further examination of the vascular system revealed no evidence of disease. A colleague from the vascular surgery department referred the patient to our consultation. When the patient presented to our clinic, she was in sheer despair. Compression treatment and consistent lymphatic drainage were unable to achieve any significant improvement.

On the day of the examination, body weight was 98 kg with a height of 1.67 m. The examination showed clinically a very pronounced lipedema of type IV stage 2.

We talked to the patient about the possible options and showed her the advantages and disadvantages and risks of surgical and conservative treatment. First, we filed an application for cost coverage, which was rejected by several instances. The patient did not want to take legal action because of the poor prospects of success.

Our surgical treatment plan included liposuction of the front of the lower extremity (hips, thighs, knee region, and lower legs) and liposuction of the back of the lower extremity. In another session, liposuction of the arms (upper arms and forearms) was also planned. If there was tissue sagging in the inner thigh area, a thigh lift could be considered (this was unlikely at the time). In addition, the patient wanted liposuction of the abdomen and flank region (we combined this with liposuction of the arms).

Finally, the planned procedures were performed (with the exception of the thigh lift). During the three liposuction procedures, nearly 28 L of fat were removed using our own technique. After each of the procedures, the patient stayed with us in the clinic for 3 days. Dizziness and nausea were not reported, there was only a slight decrease in the Hb value (hemoglobin). On each of the following days, the patient was able to move freely on the ward level. Of course, there were bruises and indurated areas. Lymphatic drainage was started early, and in time the initial swelling and bruising subsided.

The further course was unspectacular. The soft tissues recovered well. The pain was already virtually gone after the first liposuction in the surgical regions—as it was at the end of the treatments. The pain was completely gone. The patient gave up compression only slowly after 6 months. The aesthetic result was very good (for the patient and also from our point of view). The patient thanked us with a basket of chocolates at the end of the treatment. Another control will follow in 1 year.

3.9   Cost Absorption

Reimbursement for treatment, whether outpatient or inpatient, requires that the condition and treatment be recognized by the health insurance system.

Lipedema is a recognized disease and is listed as a medical diagnosis in the International Statistical Classification of Diseases and Related Health Problems (ICD).

In the German version of the current ICD-10, lipedema is coded E88.2x.

Classification according to ICD-10-GM.

E88.20 Lipedema stage I (Fig. 3.43 left)

E88.21 Lipedema stage II (Fig. 3.43 center)

E88.22 Lipedema stage III (Fig. 3.43 right)

E88.28 Other or unspecified lipedema

Thus, one part of the requirement for cost coverage is met. The other part, namely the treatment, is somewhat more problematic in this case. Conservative treatment in the sense of compression treatment and lymphatic drainage are usually covered by health insurance for life. Unfortunately, when it comes to liposuction, the situation is different. Liposuction (liposuction) is not recognized as a measure for the treatment of diseases and thus also of lipedema.

To test the effectiveness, the Federal Joint Committee (G-BA) has commissioned a clinical trial in which liposuction (surgical liposuction) has been compared with the standard nonsurgical treatment of lipedema since the beginning of 2020. During the trial study, the costs of liposuction will be borne by the statutory health insurance funds.

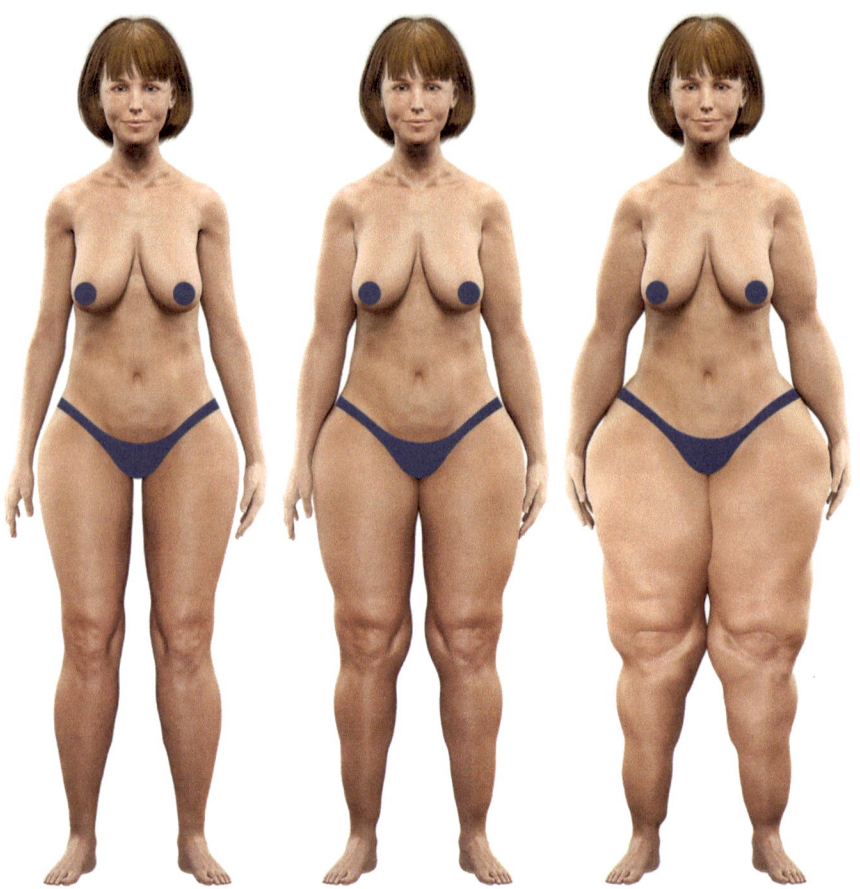

Fig. 3.43 Stages of lipedema

Women with lipedema in all stages (I–III) in the leg region can participate in the study. The basic prerequisite for participation is that there has not been sufficient relief of symptoms under conservative measures. There are a number of inclusion and exclusion criteria that we do not wish to discuss further here, as the inclusion deadline is Dec. 31, 2019. The aim of the trial study is to assess the potential of the method in the indication to include the method in the benefits catalog of the statutory health insurance (SHI) if the result is positive—a ray of hope for all patients who cannot participate in the trial study. We ourselves are participating as a study center, but we strongly criticize the study design. Through the study, we all hope to gain more insight into the extent to which liposuction has a positive effect on the symptoms of lipedema.

However, there are two other options through which liposuction is possible as a health insurance benefit.

- Since 2020, liposuction in severe cases has become a statutory health insurance benefit. By "in severe cases" it means the presence of stage III. We have already discussed in detail that this criterion makes no sense, because stage III says nothing about the pain, nor about the suffering pressure, nor any other form of impairment. The fact that stage III liposuction has been included in SHI-accredited care was decided by the Federal Joint Committee (G-BA). The service has been included for a limited period until December 31, 2024. By then, the findings from the above-mentioned trial study, which is to assess the effect of liposuction in all stages of lipedema, should be available.
- Cost absorption by the health insurance fund is also possible via a so-called individual case decision. The individual case decision is an administrative act based on separate circumstances. An individual case decision is requested from the health insurance fund. An application includes a medical report and an initially informal request formulated by you. As with all measures for which the health insurance fund is to cover the costs, there must be a medical indication.

Surely you have already read the term "medical indication" and if this is not the case, you will certainly encounter it in the course of the application process. Indication in itself means "indication of cure." It simply means which measure, for example, an operation or a drug, is the right one for the therapy of disease. The word "medical" means that the treatment is for an actual illness.

In the case of lipedema, pain or restriction of movement would be the reason for treatment. The treatment of facial wrinkles with Botox® (botulinum toxin A) or by a facelift would be a cosmetic (=aesthetic) indication, since there is no physical or health impairment here. Consequently, it is a treatment of a condition which, by definition, is not a disease. These treatments are also referred to as IGeL services (individual health services).

A medical indication exists in the case of a disease or disfigurement within the meaning of the Fifth Social Code (SGB V). This means that the health insurance fund will bear the costs of treatment for those affected. This means that in the case of a medical indication, the health insurance fund must bear the treatment costs.

Actually, the health insurance company would have to cover the costs of treatment per se, provided that the doctor sees a pathological change. Before an eye, intestinal, or foot operation, the health insurance company is not asked either, since no one gets the idea that these could be "desired operations." This is different for lipedema or tightening operations. Here, the view of the health insurance companies often differs from that of the plastic surgeons who provide a medical indication. The health insurance companies very often refuse to reimburse the treatment costs after the treatment has taken place. The health insurance company argues that there was no pathological condition and that the operations were scheduled, not acute. Therefore, the health insurer should have been asked in advance whether, in its opinion, there was a medical indication and the operation could be charged to the health insurer.

Against this background, the individual case application for cost coverage must be made in advance. Since many employees at health insurance companies are pure clerks and do not have the competence to assess medical facts, the health insurance company often helps itself with the medical service of the health insurance company (MDK).

The Medical Service of the Health Insurance Fund (MDK) is an institution that advises health insurance funds on medical issues, among other things. Doctors from various specialities are permanently employed by the Medical Service and, to put it simply, work as "experts." In the rarest of cases, the MDK can call on the services of a plastic surgeon. Therefore, doctors from other fields often deal with plastic surgery issues, which unfortunately often leads to incomprehensible decisions. But here, too, the MDK and the physicians work continuously to achieve comprehensible decisions.

Thus, health insurance usually decides only after obtaining an expert opinion from the MDK. The MDK either decides on the basis of files, which is very difficult in the case of these operations, or it conducts an expert opinion.

When are you entitled to have costs covered? Section 7 sentence 1 of the German Social Code Book V states: "Insured persons are entitled to health treatment if it is necessary in order to recognize or cure an illness, to prevent its aggravation or to alleviate symptoms of illness."

▶   Specialist lawyer T. Werner has written the very interesting Chap. 6
        with all the necessary information on medical indications and questions
        of cost coverage. I can only warmly recommend this to you.

In the case of psychological problems, according to case law, treatment with psychotherapy, or psychiatry is indicated as a priority. Therefore, you should never apply for cost coverage on the basis of psychological stress; a rejection would be inevitable.

In reality, medical indications are far less tangible than the legal text would suggest. The assessments by the MDK are so varied that we can no longer even make a prognosis as to whether costs will be covered. This most often has to do with the existing or lacking qualification of the physicians of the medical service in this particular field. How well trained is a trauma surgeon, internist, or gynecologist to decide if liposuction is the right treatment? We have read very questionable and astonishing decisions by the MDK in our daily clinical practice. In addition, the health insurance company does not always follow the recommendation of the MDK, which it does not have to per se.

Costs for operations for which there is no medical justification are not covered by health insurance. These are essentially aesthetic operations. The person concerned must pay for these. In contrast to medically justified operations, where the entire treatment, including treatment of complications, is fully covered by the health insurance, the affected person will share in the costs of complications after aesthetic operations, depending on their income. To exclude this risk of co-payment, a so-called follow-up cost insurance can be concluded. In addition, operations that are not medically indicated are charged with VAT.

▶   Medically justified interventions are operations whose costs are charged to the health insurance companies. Aesthetic procedures (operations without medical indication) are charged to the patient. The costs of follow-up operations or complications must then be borne by the patient. To avoid this risk, a special follow-up insurance policy can be taken out for this purpose before the operation.

After the refusal of cost coverage or if there is no medical indication, liposuction can also be performed as a self-pay service. The costs of liposuction depend on the number of regions to be treated during the operation as well as the difficulty of the operation, form of anesthesia, duration of anesthesia, length of stay, visits, and follow-up checks. It also plays a role whether the treatment is outpatient or inpatient in the hospital. Liposuction starts at about 1000 euros plus VAT with local anesthesia and a small circumscribed area. A hip–thigh liposuction on an outpatient basis under twilight sleep anesthesia costs about 4500–6500 Euro plus VAT. For extensive liposuction of the hip, thigh, and lower leg region, costs between 5500 and 7500 Euro plus VAT have to be calculated.

Other costs that are added to a self-pay service are follow-up insurance. If a complication occurs during a self-pay service, your health insurance company may charge you a share of the costs or refuse to cover the costs altogether. With follow-up cost insurance, you can protect yourself against this financial risk.

3.10   Autologous Fat Grafting

Angel Pecorelli Capozzi, Zaher Jandali
You may think that this chapter is rather unusual for a lipedema book. However, we performautologous fat grafting in about every tenth lipedema treatment. This corresponds to about 10% of cases and is not entirely insignificant.

Liposuctioned fat can be used very well for autologous fat grafting. Autologous fat grafting is also called "lipofilling."

▶   Autologous fat grafting is also called lipofilling.

In this process, the extracted fat is washed, processed, and transplanted. The self-transplanted fat grows on site to about 70% and remains in place forever. About 30% of the fat cells die after transplantation.

▶   In autologous fat grafting, the extracted fat is washed, processed, and transplanted.

For several years, autologous fat grafting (autologous fat transfer, lipofilling) has enjoyed increasing popularity. Most often, autologous fat transplantation is used for volume augmentation and tissue rejuvenation. Volume augmentation is often performed for breast augmentation in cases of congenital or acquired volume deficiency. When we talk about an acquired volume deficit in the breast area, we are talking about changes in the breast that occur due to the natural aging process, or weight loss. However, volume loss also occurs in the face during the aging process, as well as aging and sagging of the skin. The loss of volume in the face occurs due to a reduction of fatty tissue and bone, as well as sagging of the soft tissues due to gravity.

Over the years, various synthetic fillers and implants have been used to treat these volume deficits. Each of the substances had its advantages and disadvantages, and the practitioners always had to make compromises due to the often not insignificant disadvantages. In the past, liposuction procedures were traumatic, and fat cells were destroyed during liposuction. This is no longer the case today. Nowadays, liposuction procedures, whether WAL, PAL, or standard, are very gentle procedures and the fat cells obtained as a result have good vitality. As a result, fatty tissue has proven to be an ideal filler for the above-mentioned indications. But not only that: fatty tissue offers much more. As we have read in the introductory chapters, we also find stem cells and growth factors in adipose tissue. We can extract these stem cells and growth factors and deliver them to the skin to support collagen synthesis, improve blood circulation and improve skin quality. Here we are already in the middle of the topic of regenerative medicine. However, we most often use lipofilling for breast augmentation and wrinkle treatment.

▶ Possible applications are own fat breast augmentation, facial wrinkle treatment, lip modeling, and many more.

Autologous fat grafting is divided into two parts. First, liposuction is performed, followed by fat grafting. In all techniques, the suctioned fat must be collected in a special canister or system for fat grafting (Fig. 3.44).

After repeated cleaning and, if necessary, processing of the fatty tissue, it is drawn up into syringes and can be injected into the recipient area, for example, the breast (Fig. 3.45).

Roughly speaking, we distinguish between three types of fat that are suitable for transplantation: In addition to macro fat, which is the simple fat that we harvest with our suction cannulas, there is also micro fat and nano fat. The macro fat, as shown in Fig. 3.46, we use, for example, for breast or buttock augmentation, but also the correction of dents or irregularities. In macro fat, the fat particles are larger than 1.5 mm, on average about 2–3 or 4 mm. The fat tissue is obtained with fine cannulas.

▶ Roughly speaking, we distinguish three types of fat for autologous fat grafting: macro fat, micro fat, and nano fat.

Fig. 3.44 The collected grease is drawn up from the collection container via syringes

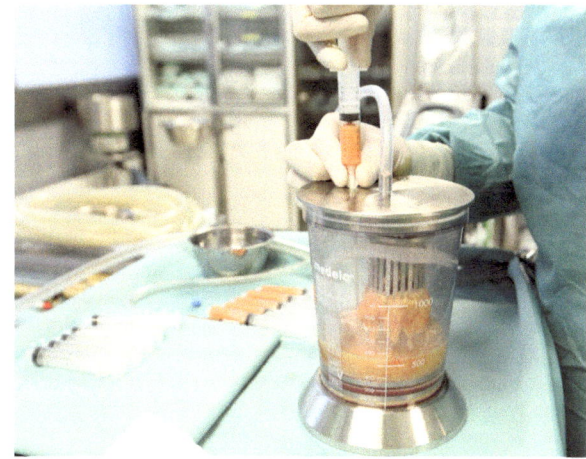

Fig. 3.45 Drawn-up fat syringes for transplantation

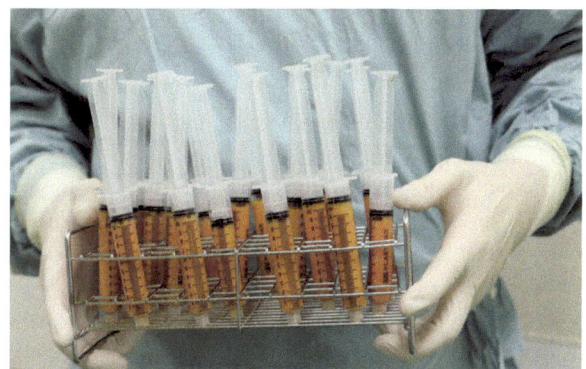

Fig. 3.46 Macro fat when inserted into the breast for breast augmentation

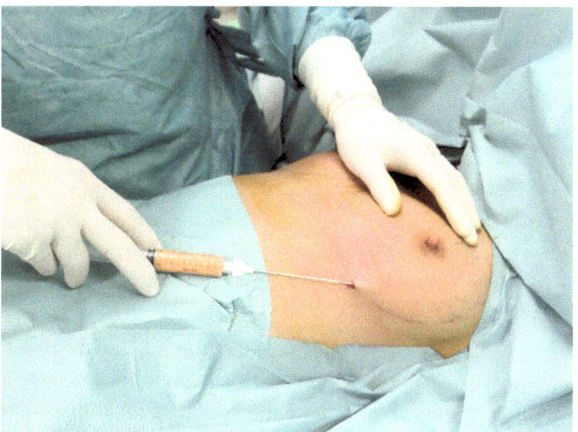

Fig. 3.47 After autologous fat grafting to the breast with previously severe asymmetry and bilateral hypovolemia

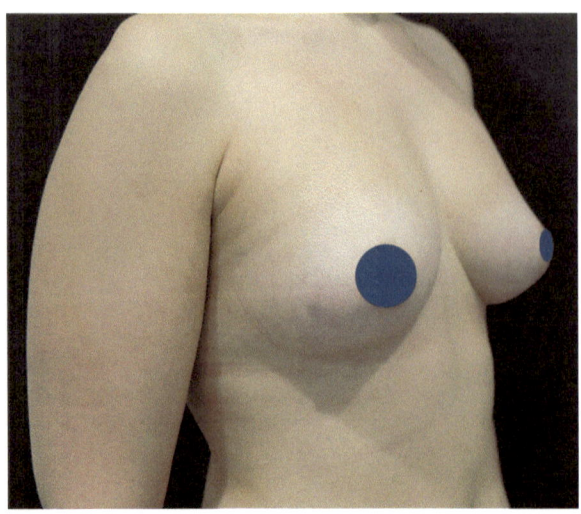

If the fat conglomerates are broken up, then we obtain micro fat (Fig. 3.47). The micro fat particles have a diameter of about 1 mm and are aspirated through special micro fat cannulas with a hole diameter of 1 mm. The micro fat is particularly suitable for facial wrinkle treatment.

When we talk about nano fat, we are basically no longer talking about adipose tissue per se, but only about the stem cells found in adipose tissue. Nano fat is all about regenerative medicine. Nano fat is produced via a process in which we first break up the fat conglomerates into tiny particles and finally further process the entire fat emulsion through a filter. In the end, we have an aqueous-yellowish emulsion that no longer contains intact fat cells, but instead contains a great many stem cells with regenerative potential. We use nano fat most frequently for sustainable improvement of the skin's appearance (Fig. 3.48).

The exact mechanism of fat cell survival after transplantation is not yet fully understood. We would like to briefly present one of the common theories: After the fat cells are removed from the donor region and transplanted into the recipient region, a race against time begins for each individual fat cell - death versus survival. For the survival of the transplanted fat cell, the supply of oxygen and nutrients is indispensable. Since the fat cells do not have their own blood vessels, they must be supplied via diffusion until the fat cells have reconnected to the local vascular network and can be nourished via it. This diffusion provides an initially sufficient supply for most of the cells.

It should be noted that the higher the oxygen content of the recipient tissue, the better the growth rate of the fat cells. Negative influencing factors such as smoking and excessive pressure on the cells should therefore be strictly avoided. Clinically, an average survival rate of transplanted fat cells of about 60–70% is observed.

▶   Autologous fat grafting in smokers more often shows a poor fat cell attachment rate. Poorer tissue perfusion and a lower oxygen supply in the recipient tissue are responsible for this.

Fig. 3.48 Micro and nano grease

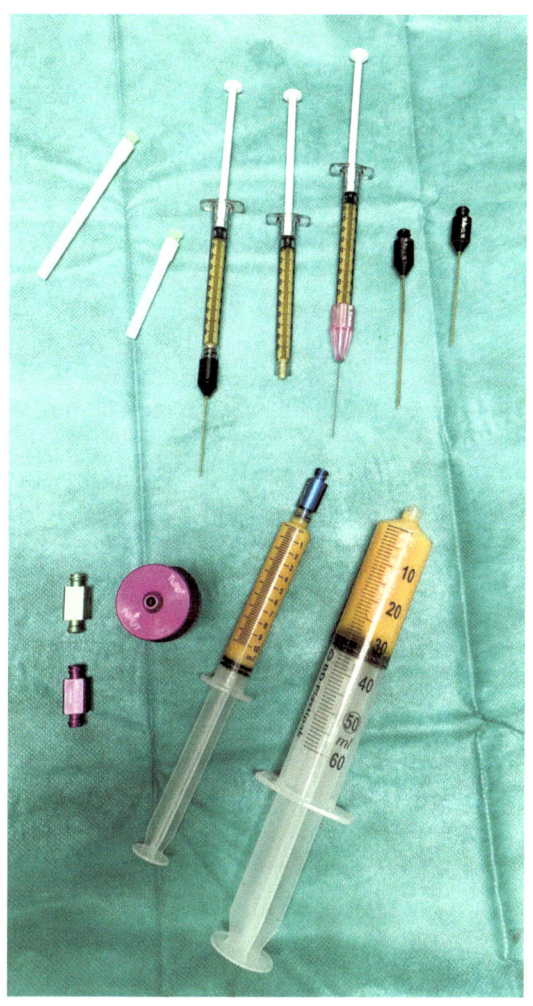

In addition, it is important to avoid too much pressure on the transplanted area. Pressure from the outside causes reduced blood flow, which in turn causes the cells to die. This means, for example, that you should not wear a compression bra or tight bandage at first after a breast augmentation. You can wear a light sports bra that does not exert much pressure from the second week. Likewise, you should not lie on your stomach after a breast augmentation with your own fat. Too much internal pressure due to "overfilling" with fat cells can also lead to fat cell death. Warmth, on the other hand, has a positive effect on fat cell survival. The warmer the recipient area, the better the blood circulation in this area.

The most important factor for the growth of as many fat cells as possible is the technique of transplantation. If fat transplantation is performed with an excessive amount of fat tissue, too much internal pressure is exerted on the transplanted cells. On the one hand, this impairs the blood supply to the resident cells, and on the other hand, the diffusion necessary to supply nutrients to the transplanted cells is impaired, so that both groups of cells may die.

For the reasons just mentioned, fat grafting to the breast, for example, can sometimes be performed with only 100 mL, sometimes with up to 400 mL or more per breast. So how much fat can be transplanted depends on how much well perfused, localized tissue is available. If you naturally have little subcutaneous fat in the breast area, very little fat can be transplanted in the first few grafts. In this first transplantation, the surgeon creates a so-called graft store with the fat grafts for the following transplantations. If the tissue thickness in the breast is sufficiently good, a larger volume can be transplanted directly in the first procedure.

Due to the volume limitation during surgery, breast augmentation is performed, depending on the target size and in several sessions. As a rule, one to three sessions are planned. This step-by-step procedure to ensure the success of the therapy is called sequential autologous fat grafting.

The most frequently asked question when it comes to the topic of autologous fat is whether lipedema then develops in the breast with a halting growth of the fat cells. From our many years of experience, we can answer this question with a clear no. If, for example, breast augmentation has been performed using autologous fat transplantation, the breast will behave quite naturally afterwards. If you gain weight, the breast volume increases. If you lose weight, the breast volume decreases. Painful breasts after autologous fat transplantation have not yet been described to us. Unfortunately, there is not enough scientific work in this area either. It also seems that the painfulness has more to do with the location of the fat cell than with the fat cell itself, which makes sense.

Body Contouring Surgery After Extensive Liposuction and Weight Loss

4

Zaher Jandali, Benedikt Merwart, and Lucian Jiga

The last component of our complex surgical treatment plan for lipedema is the treatment of any excess skin-soft tissue. In many patients, these measures are not necessary, however, in certain cases, there is a medical indication for body shape restoration. This is especially true for patients with stage 3 (or according to our classification +++) or with massive weight loss associated with lipedema. The most common surgical corrections in such patients are the thigh and upper arm lifts, but also abdominoplasty, circular torso, and buttock lifts.

4.1 Medical Indication for Tightening of Excess Skin and Soft Tissues

A medical indication for treatment exists in the case of a specific disease or disfigurement. This means that the health insurance must or should bear the treatment costs.

Skin irritation is the most frequently expressed complaint. Heat accumulates due to skin surfaces lying on top of each other, and in the absence of air circulation, moist chamber forms, disrupting the natural skin barrier. This favors the formation of chronic open wounds with fungal and bacterial infections. These are usually found in the area of the inner thighs, armpits, and the fold of the abdominal wall. The continuous rubbing taking place in these areas can lead to real sores and pain and can be responsible for the use of pain medication.

The excess "skin flaps," especially on the upper arms and thighs (Fig. 4.1), result in a restriction of natural movement in everyday life and especially during sport. The excessive soft tissues and skin will lag behind at each arm and leg movement

Z. Jandali (✉) · B. Merwart · L. Jiga
Department of Plastic, Aesthetic, Reconstructive and Hand Surgery, Evangelical Hospital Oldenburg, Oldenburg, Niedersachsen, Germany
e-mail: dr@jandali.de

Fig. 4.1 Lipedema after massive weight loss with the emerging need for tightening surgery

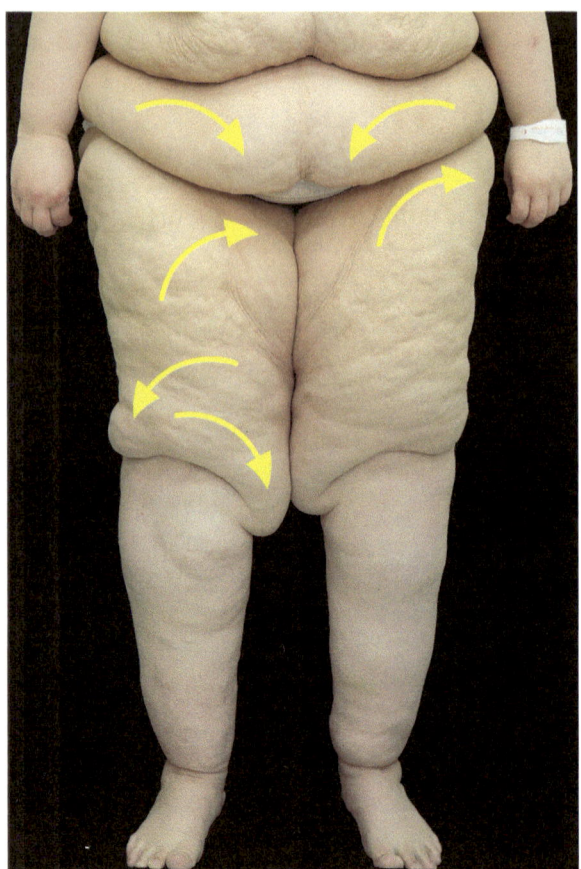

due to their inherent inertia. Here, the restrictions range from "somewhat disturbing," which certainly cannot be applied as a justification for a medical indication, to "I can hardly move" or "sport is not possible per se." The chronic sweating and the associated unpleasant body odor lead to social withdrawal and the feeling of stigmatization.

4.2 Noninvasive and Minimally Invasive Tightening Methods

Before we discuss different tightening operations in the following sections, we would like to take a brief look at alternatives to surgical skin tightening. For some time now, there have been various devices on the market that can be used for noninvasive tightening. We distinguish here the devices that act on the skin and connective tissue from the surface of the body, after liposuction from the devices that are inserted into the tissue through an incision through the skin and act directly on the tissue. These two different approaches are called "noninvasive "when acting from the outside and "invasive "when acting directly from the inside.

Invasive devices applied following liposuction use the same small incisions through which liposuction was performed. Therefore, these devices are also referred to as "minimally invasive" in their application.

What they all have in common is a transfer of energy to the collagen fiber network of the connective tissue, causing it to shrink and thus achieving a tightening effect. In Fig. 4.2 we show such a shrinking process.

You are probably wondering what we mean by energy transfer"? Ultimately, it is the heat above 50 C at the depth that causes denaturation, dehydration, and collagen contracture (collagen shrinkage) in the connective tissue. Of these mechanisms, collagen shrinkage is the most important for the tightening effect.

It should be noted that devices that are applied from the body surface have a significantly lower effect than devices that act directly in the tissue. The reasons are the long distance from the body surface to the connective tissue and the much poorer dosage of energy delivery into the tissue.

Noninvasive devices mostly work with ultrasound, laser, or radiofrequency. The effect is rather limited to the superficial tissue layers. Invasive devices with laser, radiofrequency current, or helium plasma also have a limited range of effects, but because they are used in the tissue, treatment of the deep tissue parts can be carried out well.

The market is full of devices, and there are many more types of devices, which are due to their abundancy will not be elaborated further in this chapter. All these devices are limited in their effect and are not miracle weapons against skin sagging. Within these devices, we distinguish medical from cosmetic devices.

Cosmetic devices are all noninvasive and freely available to everyone . They are devices with which it is very difficult to cause harm, regardless of the method of application. Such cosmetic devices can be found at beauticians and beauty salons.

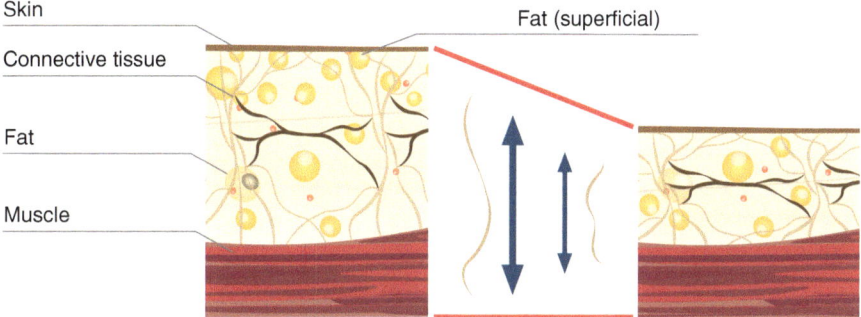

Fig. 4.2 Shrinkage of collagen fibers

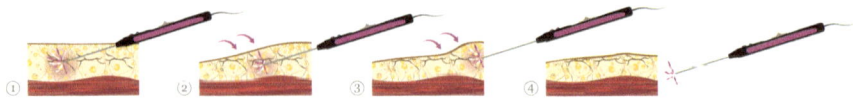

Fig. 4.3 Function of the helium plasma beam

Medical devices have a completely different depth of penetration and may usually only be used by the physician himself or, more rarely, under medical supervision or guidance. What does this mean? If a device is difficult to cause damage, the effect cannot be very great either. For this reason, after treatment with cosmetic devices, you often see no effect at all or only a very small effect, which in most cases does not correspond to what you and we would like to see. Conversely, medical devices that can achieve a great effect also carry a certain risk of causing tissue damage. At this point, it should be added that even among medical devices, there are many that have limited effects or are of no good at all.

We do not recommend treatment with cosmetic devices if a proper tightening effect is desired. We also advise caution with medical devices, as they often do not provide the desired result.

One of the most promising methods is the use of a helium plasma beam immediately following liposuction. In this case, the liposuction is first performed as usual, and at the end of the operation, a probe is inserted into the tissue through the small incisions of the suction. As with other methods, energy is transferred in the form of heat to the connective tissue and collagen fibers. In the helium plasma technique, it is the helium plasma jet that transfers the energy in the form of heat. The helium plasma device works in cycles. One cycle of tissue heating and cooling lasts about 0.75 s, and the helium plasma beam is triggered for only 0.044 s thereby heating the tissue to a temperature of up to 85 °C. This punctual high temperature ensures the effects of tissue shrinkage described above are achieved. The principle of the helium plasma beam is illustrated in Fig. 4.3.

4.3   Conclusion

We do not recommend a noninvasive method after liposuction. Since the energy does not arrive where it should, the noninvasive method does not make sense in most cases.

A series of liposuctions involving over 20 l of aspirate in the legs will certainly result in the desire for a tightening procedure. However in such instances, in the presence of significant loose skin areas minimally invasive techniques will not bring much in terms of tissue tightening.

Keep in mind that many devices out there are not good. Before you throw your money out the window, you should carefully consider which therapy is the most suitable for your problem. We are currently testing various systems so we do not yet want to make any recommendations, although the helium plasma method looks very promising.

4.4 Thigh Lift

Do you suffer from sagging skin of the inner thighs always rubbing against each other, becomes red and sore, after lipedema treatment? Then you probably belong to the group of patients who are thinking about a thigh lift. Despite sports, massages, and compression treatment, the skin in the thigh area often does not regress sufficiently. Unfortunately, a lasting tightening of the thighs can often only be achieved through surgery.

If complaints are present, in Germany the costs for a thigh lift are covered by health insurance. Typical complaints are an annoying excess of soft tissue (skin) on the inner sides of the thighs, on the inner sides of the knees, and areas above the knees as well as the transition to the lower legs.

Especially on the inner thighs, the rubbing against each other of the skin excess generates wounds very reluctant to treatment, an understandable fact due to the constant movement in this area. Often, the soft tissues also become painfully trapped in the pants or underwear. Not to be neglected is the self or subjectively detectable disfigurement of the body shape.

A good prerequisite for a thigh lift is approximately normal body weight, preferably not overweight. The less subcutaneous fat tissue is present, the better the tightening can be performed, the lower the operative risk and the better the result.

In the case of the thighs, we also distinguish between pure sagging of the skin and sagging of the skin in combination with fat pads that are still present (Fig. 4.4). Depending on the extent of the excess, there are different techniques that can be used to optimally address this problem. These have undergone continuous development in recent years in spite of previously documented complications such as wound healing disorders, lymphatic vessel injuries, etc.

Meanwhile, most thigh lifts are prepared via liposuction, or at least liposuction is one major part of the treatment concept. In the authors' clinics, a thigh lift without liposuction is virtually out of the question. Adequate thinning of tissues through lipoaspiration avoids deep tissue incisions and the consecutive risks of wound healing problems, infections, and lymphatic injuries.

In principle, we distinguish between a pure groin incision and a vertical incision in the inner thigh area as well as a combination of both. Via the pure groin incision, only excess in the inner upper area of the thighs can be tightened. If the excess extends beyond the middle third of the inner thigh towards the feet or in case of extensive sagging, an additional vertical incision should be made.

The thigh lift is clearly separate from the buttock lift, but both can be combined. Unlike the thigh lift, the buttock lift involves an incision in the fold of the buttock envelope, through which the buttocks are tightened. Although the scar or incision of the thigh lift ends in the gluteal fold, it does not tighten the buttocks as well.

Procedure

Before the operation, the surgeon makes a drawing. Photos are also taken for documentation and the important incision lines are marked. Figure 4.5 shows a typical drawing before a thigh lift. The blue markings for liposuction vary depending on the

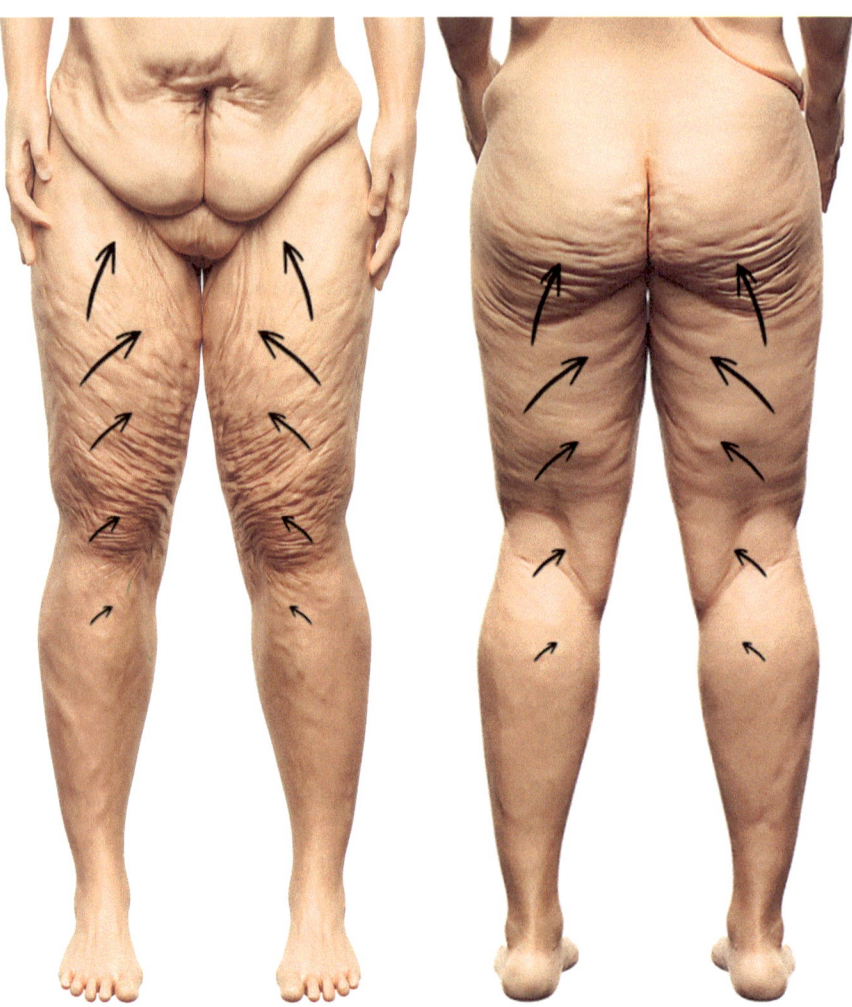

Fig. 4.4 Sagging skin on the thighs

initial situation, cost transfer from the health insurance company and the necessity for the lift. The areas to be removed are marked in red. The black lines mark the expected scars.

On the day of surgery, after induction of anesthesia, a "special saline solution" is injected in the interest areas using an automatic pump as preparation for liposuction. Subsequently, liposuction mainly of the inner sides, but usually beyond these, the front sides and outer sides are performed. This is done to shape a harmonic transition between the areas to be tightened and the adjacent thigh regions.

In the past, an incision was made in the groin and vertically on the thigh without prior liposuction. If excess fatty tissue was still present, this was removed directly through the incision. However, the problem was that such cutting away of

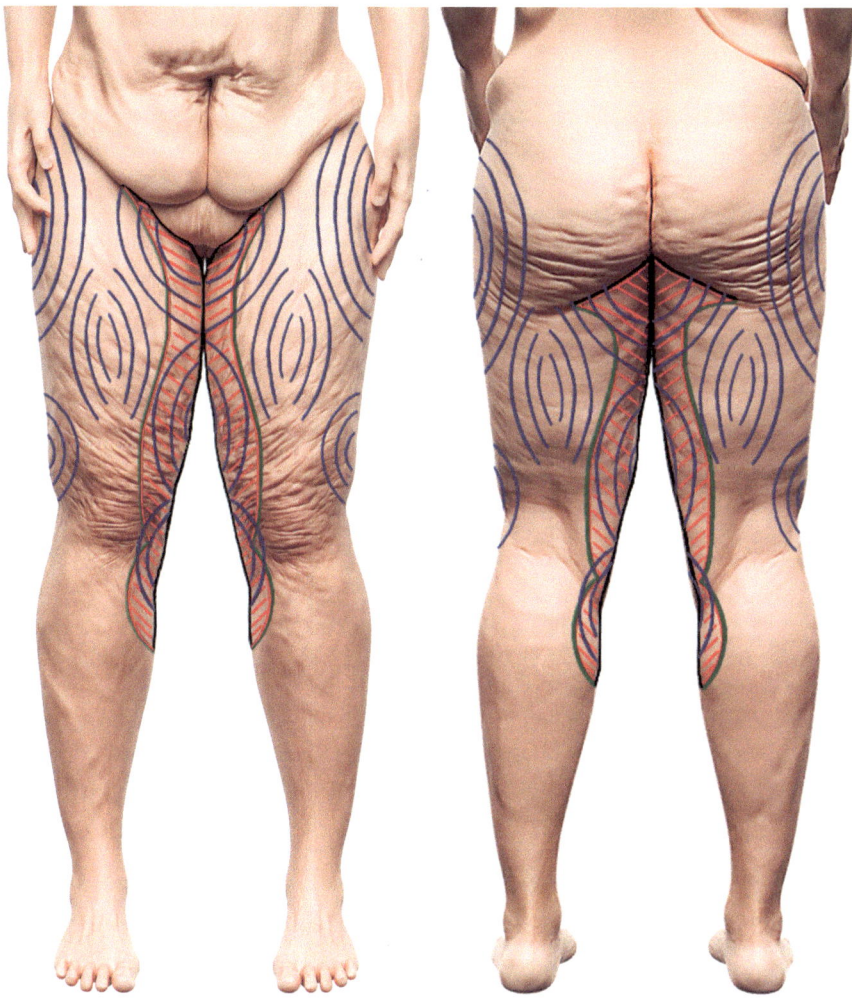

Fig. 4.5   Plan drawing of a thigh lift before surgery

tissue left a much deeper unsightly incision and subsequent scar than is the case with the liposuction method. It is precisely these deep incisions that often result in injury to lymphatic vessels and other structures such as blood vessels. If infection occurred in these situations—and the thigh lift has an increased risk of infection anyway due to the localization (anogenital)—these were relatively extensive and severe.

From all the above, it is clear why we regularly prepare the lifting through liposuction. Liposuction is performed thoroughly and extensively so that only a small amount of fat remains. In the next step, the excess skin is removed—depending on the planned incision either only in the groin or starting at the level of the knees up to the groin. In the area of the inner thighs, the skin is removed quite superficially, so that even the deep layer of skin (dermis) is often left in place. The soft tissues are then folded in, intertwined, and sutured.

When an incision is made in the groin, it is also made superficially to avoid lymphatic injury, but it cannot be made quite as superficially in the groin as in the thigh area. Here, too, deeper incisions were made in the past, and unwanted complications were common.

In the case of very pronounced skin sagging, the soft tissues of the thighs are suspended with so-called inner anchor sutures on the pelvis during the operation. The function of these anchor sutures is to maintain the tightening effect and prevent the inner thigh soft tissues from sinking due to gravity. Usually, one to two drains are inserted into the wound for drainage of wound secretions.

The skin incision is closed using modern suture materials. All skin sutures are self-dissolving. In addition, a skin adhesive or staple plaster is applied to the skin suture. This has the advantage of further sealing the wound against germs in the genital region. After the application of a dressing, compression pants are applied. The compression pants applied in the operating room must be worn consistently for 8 weeks. The inpatient hospital stay lasts between 2 and 5 days.

Figure 4.6 shows a thigh lift with a T incision and liposuction before and after as a scheme. Real results may differ.

In painless patients, lymphatic drainage can be initiated soon after surgery. In case of pains, postponing lymphatic drainage for a few days is recommended.

On the day of the operation you may already get up, but very few patients feel able to do so and do not get up until 1 day after the operation. The first time you get up, you should always be accompanied by a specialist nurse.

We recommend physical rest for 6–8 weeks depending on the extent of the operation. During the first 3 weeks, we recommend lying at home more and not overexerting yourself. Sports should be taken up after 8 weeks at the earliest.

After a thigh lift, our patients ask for pain medication more often than after other operations. Nevertheless, such pains are kept within limits.

Once the drains have been removed, showering is allowed. In any case, showers should be kept short so as not to soak the wounds and thus minimize the risk of impaired wound healing. The scars should initially be blow-dried dry after showering or bathing.

Complications and Risks
Particular risks of a thigh lift are:

- Wound healing disorders.
- Injury to lymphatic vessels (lymphedema).
- Accumulation of wound fluid.
- Wounds that tear open.
- Scars that have healed unfavorably.
- slight asymmetries.

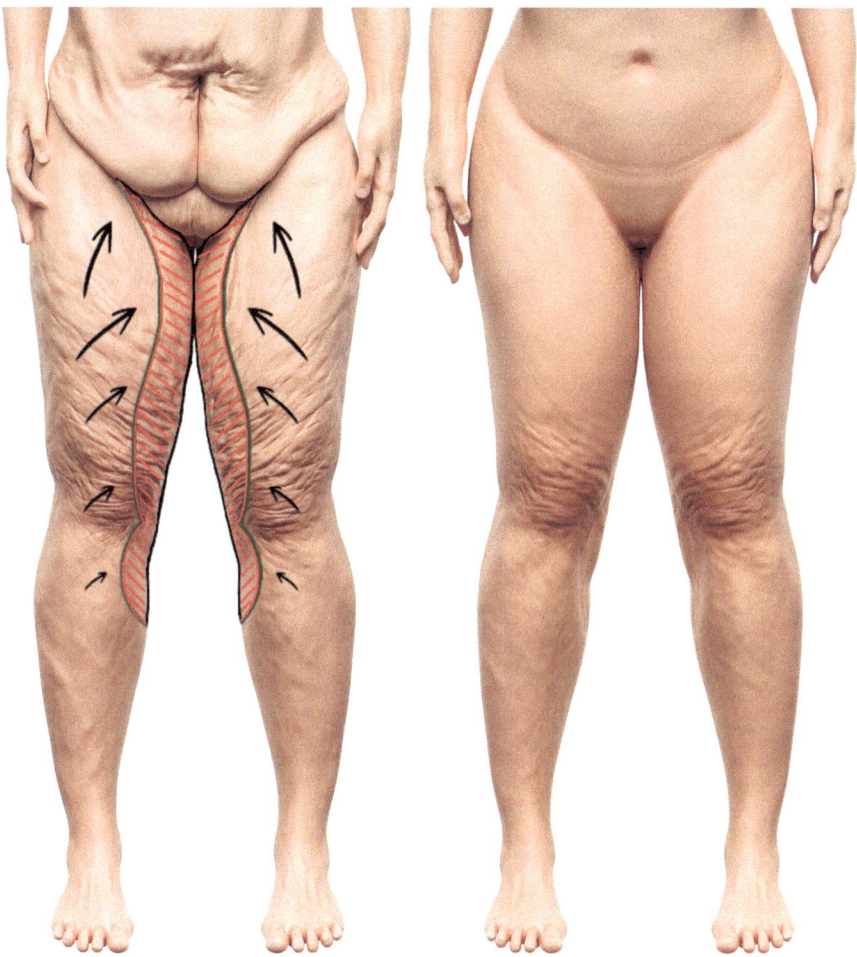

Fig. 4.6 Plan drawing of a thigh lift before surgery

Other risks will be discussed in detail during the consultation with your treating physician.

If a thigh lift is performed at the patient's own expense, costs of 3500–8500 euros plus VAT can be expected (Fig. 4.7).

▷   A thigh lift is an operation that is sometimes accompanied by large scars. The extent of the scars should be shown to you before the treatment by means of before and after pictures. To treat thighs with significant excess skin in the long term, a thigh lift is the only good option.

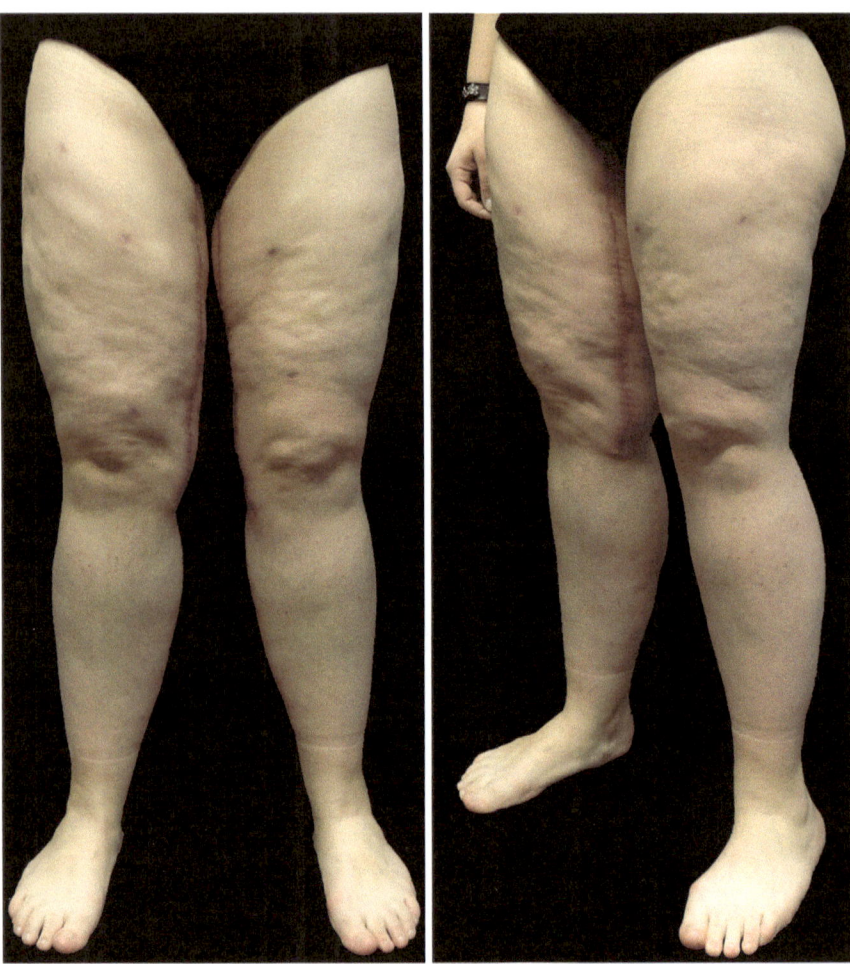

Fig. 4.7 Result after thigh lift surgery

4.5   Upper Arm Lift

Sagging and excess skin on the upper arms are often not only aesthetically disturbing but can also lead to functional discomfort and everyday restriction. We see sagging upper arms less often than sagging thighs after extensive liposuction for lipedema. Thus, the desire for an upper arm lift is also somewhat less common among lipedema sufferers than the desire for a thigh lift. The more pronounced the lipedema, the more skin must regress under its own power (Fig. 4.8).

Perhaps you also suffer from sagging skin on the upper arms. Then you know very well that sagging excess skin on the upper arms can really cause problems. Many people think, "Oh, sagging skin on the upper arms, it doesn't matter!" This is not true. Most often, patients complain that the excess skin on the upper arms

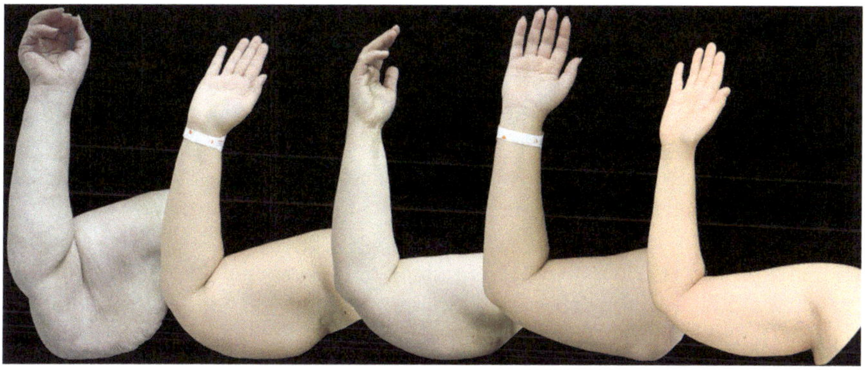

Fig. 4.8 Different manifestations in the different stages of lipedema (before liposuction)

interferes with the natural flow of movement, making it impossible to move easily in everyday life, not to mention sports. If the excess already interferes with everyday life, sports are usually out of the question.

But we are also talking about extreme manifestations because we distinguish between mild, moderate, severe, and extreme excesses. Often, as those affected with pronounced excess describe it, the soft tissues hit the back of a chair, causing bruising and painful hardening. There is also often pinching and constriction of the skin, especially of the upper arm extensions toward the armpit, even with normal width clothing. These pinchings are felt by the patients as very painful, which is absolutely understandable. Likewise, the soft tissues on the chest wall and in the armpit chafe with consequently painful sores. Furthermore, there is notable inertia of the excess during movement, especially if fat tissue is still present. This is a particular problem with the arms.

After liposuctions, usually only a pure excess of skin is observed on the upper arms with or without continuation to the armpit and with only small or few fat excesses. In such a situation, it is recommended to perform a pure skin tightening operation (= upper arm lift), possibly with extension to the chest wall/armpit (=extended upper arm lift). For fine contouring, liposuction can be used if necessary, which we. We almost always perform this on the transitions to the forearm.

An upper arm lift can be performed as an outpatient or inpatient procedure, depending on the extent of the surgery. Pure liposuction generally remains on an outpatient basis. In most cases, we perform the actual upper arm lift under inpatient conditions and a stay of 2–3 days, as we usually tighten the upper arms, armpit, and, if necessary, part of the lateral chest wall. However, circumscribed upper arm lifts that do not extend beyond the arms are also well suited for outpatient treatment.

Procedure

The inpatient admission takes place on the day of the operation. As with all plastic surgery tightening operations, we mark the patient in a standing position beforehand. Marking is done to ensure symmetry and for photographic documentation of the incision. In the process, an incision is planned on the undressed upper body from the crook of the arm to the armpit, and if necessary the lateral chest wall, until the end of the excess is reached.

The surgery can be performed under local and general anesthesia. We recommend short general anesthesia for your comfort alone . The operation is usually performed simultaneously on both sides by two surgeons, whereby the decisive steps (initial incision and determining the amount of tissue to be removed) are always performed by the main surgeon in order to ensure symmetry.

Depending on how much residual fat depot is present, more or less extensive liposuction takes place right at the beginning of the operation to remove the excess residual fat tissue in the upper arms. After liposuction, or if it is not necessary, the open part of the surgery begins with the skin incision. Subsequently, the fat tissue is either cut in depth down to the so-called upper arm fascia (connective tissue layer that separates skin and fat tissue from muscles and the important vascular-nerve bundles) or we perform a purely superficial skin removal. The choice of procedure depends on how much fatty tissue is present. If possible, the fascia should not be injured, because immediately below the fascia is the important vascular-nerve bundle mentioned above, which is responsible for the blood and nerve supply of the entire arm.

Further during surgery, the excess soft tissues are detached backward as far as is necessary for the tightening. Once sufficient tightening has been achieved, the excess soft tissues are removed. During this process, the lateral uniformity is checked with a centimeter measure. The prerequisite for this is that the arms looked approximately the same before the operation. If there was a certain difference between the two arms before the operation, we assess the result by comparing the sides. The wound is closed (the suture) with self-dissolving suture material, first in a single button suture technique in the area of the dermis (the lower layer of skin) and then as a continuous suture in the epidermis.

In the first part of the operation, we first tighten only the upper arms and then move on to the armpit area to tighten the soft tissues there as well and create a smooth transition. Not always, but in most cases, one drain is inserted for each side. Don't worry: removing the drains is basically not painful; the drains are removed after the negative pressure within the tubes has been released. After adjusting the soft tissues in the armpit area, liposuction is performed at the junction of the upper and lower arm to shape the transition from the suture to the lower arm . At the end of the operation, after skin closure and applying staple plasters, either elastic wrapped or a custom-made bolero or sleeves are applied.

The operation time varies between 1 and 3 h for a complex tightening with suction. After the operation, the patient returns to the ward via the recovery room. No particular pain is reported by the patients after the operation. Tablets and possibly infusions are used to treat pain. Figure 4.9 shows an early postoperative situation after upper arm/chest wall lift and circular body lift in several surgical steps.

The arms must be protected from heavy loads for a total of 8 weeks after the operation, whereby a cautious loading can begin as early as the second or third week. You will receive more detailed information from your surgeon.

Fig. 4.9 Early postoperative picture of an upper arm lift

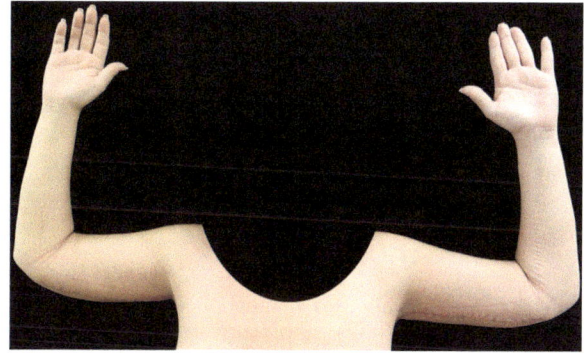

The applied sleeves should be worn continuously for 6–8 weeks. If the arms have been wrapped with an elastic bandage after surgery, a change to sleeves or a bolero should be made in the early postoperative period. Sleeves can be removed for showering and washing. The rest of the time, the sleeves should be worn continuously. For better hygiene, a second sleeve should be prescribed for all patients undergoing arm lifting.

A first shower is allowed after the removal of the drains. However, all wounds must be closed at this time. The showering should be very short, after showering the wounds should be air blow-dried. After the last wound crust falls off (2–3 weeks), scar treatment can be started with the silicone gel or silicone overlay treatment.

If you suffer from an increased tendency to sweat , the sweat glands can be removed during the operation. This is an additional service, its costs not being covered by health insurance. However, since the operation does not get significantly longer nor much complicated, the cost is kept within reasonable limits. You can discuss the details with your surgeon.

Complications and Risks

As with any surgical procedure, complications can also occur with an upper arm lift. The risks listed below, as with all other surgical descriptions, are merely an excerpt of all possible surgical risks that your attending physician will discuss with you in detail.

The specific risks of an upper arm lift are:

– Postoperative bleeding.
– Bruising.
– Infections.
– Scar breakdown.
– Wound healing disorders.

Particularly in the armpit, the wound may tear open. However, such wounds will usually heal on their own. In such situations, care must be taken to ensure that in spite of open wounds the arms are sufficiently moved so that no functional deficit remains.

Injury to the main vascular nerve bundle of the arm is a serious complication, but it is extremely unlikely.

Other risks include: Pain, swelling, bruising, tissue loss (necrosis) with revisional surgery, widened scars, asymmetry of the sides with respect to each other, remaining skin-soft tissue excess, bleeding within the surgery, deep vein thrombosis, pulmonary embolism.

▶   Especially the scars in the area of the upper arms tend to widen. The
      dermis (corium) in this area is very thin and not as strong as in other
      areas of the body. Therefore, after suturing, this layer sometimes cannot
      sufficiently keep the tension away from the top layer of skin, epidermis,
      which can result in a widened scar.

4.6   Buttock Lift

A buttock lift alone is a relatively rarely requested operation—but more frequently by lipedema patients than individuals with no lipedema after massive weight loss. First of all, for the sake of understanding, we need to distinguish upper buttock sagging from lower buttock sagging, both being usually present to a certain degree. Upper buttock sagging means that skin and soft tissues above the buttocks have sagged, causing the buttocks to droop. Deep buttock sagging means that the soft tissues are saggy, especially at the fold of the buttocks towards the thigh.

Those who actually have a lot of excess skin and tissue on the lower buttocks usually suffer from a particularly high level of distress. Perhaps you also suffer from these soft-tissue excesses on the lower buttocks? If so, you can confirm that such problems make sitting almost impossible. We have to imagine this excess of skin-soft tissue on the buttocks as if one were sitting on an unstable, flat water cushion. The exceeding skin has no stable subcutaneous connection to the deep tissue, causing a type of restless sitting with constant sliding back and forth on the buttocks. Finally, moist chambers often form within the skin folds, which aggravates into additional slippage and pain due to redness and/or pinching of the skin folds.

For upper and lower buttock sagging, different operations are recommended, possibly also a combination, because, in case of severe upper buttock sagging with buttocks hanging deeply downwards, there is almost always also a deep sagging present. Upper buttock tightening is usually performed via a circular body lift. The buttocks are lifted upward (headward) with simultaneous possible volumization (enlargement) during the same surgery if necessary, using the patient's own excess tissues. For more details, see Sect. 4.6. The lower buttock lift removes the overlapping and excess soft tissue in the area of the buttock fold. Figure 4.10 shows the initial situation before and the result after a buttock lift.

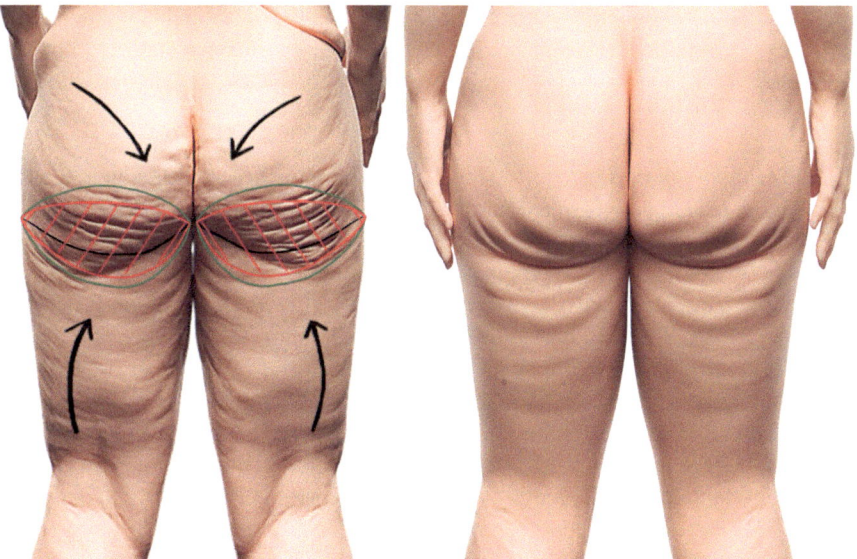

Fig. 4.10 Drawing of a buttock lift before and after surgery

4.7   Tightening of the Lower Torso Wall

Many also suffer from excess skin in the lower trunk region after losing weight to treat lipedema. Therefore, we have decided to devote a separate section to this problem.

The lower torso region is a complex interaction of several areas on the body that influence each other. Therefore, the region must also be considered in the overall picture in order to achieve a harmonious end result. Anatomically, we understand the lower torso region to be the region that begins just below the sternum, extends through the lower ribs to the pubic area and groin regions, and ends at the transition to the buttocks. The flanks (lateral region as the transition between the anterior and posterior torso wall) and thighs at the front and back are included.

You will find the recommendation as to which surgical measure or measures are necessary to correct the torso wall in your individual therapy plan. In principle, the following interventions can be distinguished from each other:

1. Fat apron removal: Here, a pure removal (we also call it resection) of the fat apron is performed without a significant tightening of the torso wall and usually without a displacement of the belly button, although sometimes with a belly button removal.
2. Abdominoplasty: A tightening of the entire anterior lower torso wall is performed through an incision from the iliac crest of one side through the pubic area to the iliac crest of the opposite side. During this procedure, the belly button is moved and, if necessary, additional liposuction of the flanks is performed to adjust the transition.

3. Circular lower body lift: Here a tightening of the abdomen, pubic region, flanks, back, and buttocks takes place. Indirectly, the thighs are also slightly tightened. Other procedures in the area of the back lower torso wall include a back lift and buttock-only lift.

Individually, these procedures should be differentiated and a treatment plan for that region should be integrated into the overall treatment plan as needed.

In the following, we will focus exclusively on the third procedure, the circular lower body lift, as this is a combination and further development of several procedures to achieve an effective tightening of the entire lower trunk region (Fig. 4.11). Via the circular body lift, in addition to the abdominal wall as the central element, the flanks, lower back or upper buttock region, and specifically the outer sides of the thighs are also tightened. Because the circular lower body lift is one of the few ways to tighten the outer sides of the thighs, it is of particular interest to those who have undergone large volume liposuction. The final step of the circular lower body lift is an abdominoplasty. We do not discuss fat apron removal; here we refer to our guidebook "Reconstructive surgery after massive weight loss," also published by Springer Medizin Verlag.

In the past, all these individual partial steps were performed over several operations. With the body lift, these can be all combined in one surgery. The body lift is particularly suitable after weight loss or after a drastic loss of volume of the flanks, thighs, and buttocks region.

The incision is circular, i.e. 360° around the entire lower part of the torso. In the area of the anterior torso wall (i.e. the abdomen), the incision is the same as the incision of an abdominoplasty, i.e. from the iliac crest of one side via the pubic region to the iliac crest of the opposite side. The incision is continued over the lateral flank

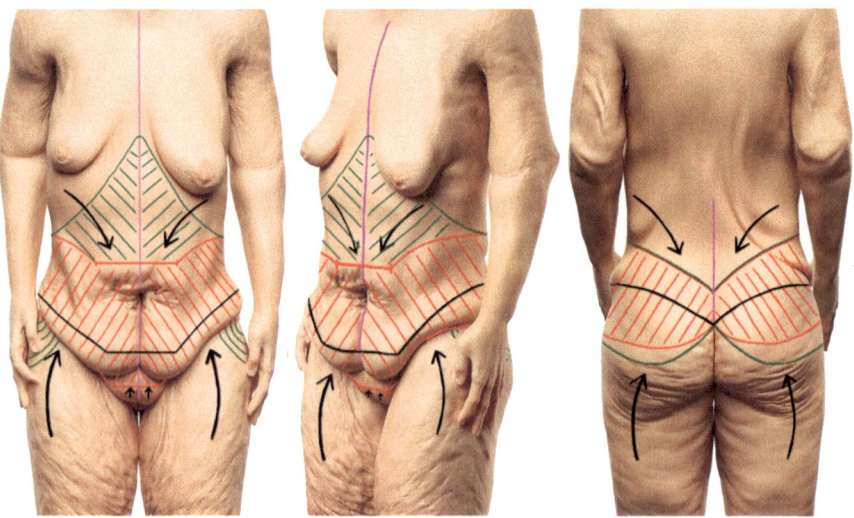

Fig. 4.11 Drawing of a buttock lift before and after surgery

region, then sloping down towards the intergluteal fold. In this way, a tightening of the abdomen, flanks, outer thighs, back, buttocks, and inner thighs can be achieved. However, the tightening of the inner thighs is only an indirect tightening, which is not performed by an incision on the inner thighs, but by tightening the subcutaneous connective tissue. Some surgeons combine the body lift with a direct thigh lift, i.e., a thigh lift with an incision on the inner thighs and/or groin. We refrain from this because in our opinion the operation then becomes too extensive and complications often arise. The scars after a circular body lift can be well concealed after healing with pants, swimsuits, or similar.

▶   Direct tightening is tightening achieved through a direct approach, i.e., tightening through an incision. Indirect tightening can be achieved without an incision from tightening of the subcutaneous connective tissue and realignment of tensile forces.

Fifteen to twenty years ago, body lifting was a very rare surgery, but with the continuous development of bariatric surgery, its indications have dramatically changed with high numbers of patients requesting body remodeling. Over time, the demand for body lifts increased accordingly.

The first body lifts—even those we performed in the beginning—were exciting and cathegorized as special operations. We operated with at least three doctors, and the patients donated 3–5 units of their own blood to replace the quite high intraoperative blood loss. The operations were challenging and lasted 6–8 h and sometimes longer. The patients stayed at least 1–2 weeks in the hospital. Fortunately, all these are history today, the body lift surgery continuously evolving into a standard operation.

As with many operations, there are also numerous different techniques for the body lift. We differentiate in our clinical everyday life two techniques, after which we perform this surgery, depending on the body image and initial conditions. Which technique will be used depends largely on the lateral thigh region. If the soft parts of the thigh hang down deeply with wrinkled skin on the outer side, we favor a technique according to Ted Lockwood, a Texas plastic surgeon, in which we can also properly correct these outer sides in particular. Here, we operate two times in the lateral position and one time in the supine position, which is why we also call it the "lateral-side-back position." What this means exactly, we will explain to you in a moment during the surgical steps. However, the most frequently performed body lift technique is a technique in which surgery begins in the prone position and ends with the abdominal wall tightening in the supine position. For this reason, we simply call it "prone position-back position."

As we said, the body lift offers many advantages and one of the main advantage is that several operations are combined in one operation . This saves you several anesthesias, you reduce the hospital stays to one, simplifying simultaneously your social life. You have only one convalescence time (recovery time after surgery) and you reduce the number of your visits to the doctor before as well as after the surgery to a considerable extent.

The most significant advantage from the plastic surgery point of view is the ability of this technique to provide if the indication is correct an optimal body shape. But what does that mean-body shapability? Let's say you want a body lift because of your body contour, and your body would actually be suitable for it: The skin and soft tissues hang on the abdomen, flanks, thighs, back, and buttocks. Now, if only the abdomen or the back alone were to be tightened, it would be difficult to achieve a really good result overall. It may even lead to a poor result because the result does not harmonize with the rest of the body image.

It is different, however, when a circular tightening can be performed. Here, a harmonious and coherent tightening of the entire lower torso wall can be achieved in one operation. This is what we mean when talking about optimal body shape. However, even this technique has its limits.

▶   A body lift is particularly suitable after weight loss in the context of lipedema treatment for a tightening of the outer thighs. The main advantage of a body lift over an abdominoplasty is that there are no dog ears at the end of the suture.

Where there are advantages, there are also disadvantages—no question about it. One of the disadvantages of a circular body lift surgery is the longer surgery time compared to the other procedures addressing each body area at a time. A body lift takes longer than an abdominoplasty, buttock lift, flank lift, or back lift. However, if trying to summarize operation times of individual surgeries and compare them with the body lift, the OR time for the latter is much shorter. However, the blood loss during the operation is higher, and the risks of anesthesia also increase due to the prolonged operation time. The recovery time after the surgery is also longer, although in total it is much shorter than the sum of all partial steps.

Experience has shown that if the bodyweight is still too high, the risk of complications of a body lift operation increases, and this cannot be justified. For BMIs of or above 30 kg/m2, we rarely perform this surgery. If you have extreme muscle mass or a high BMI despite little fat tissue, we would probably still perform the operation on you, because physical fitness is a very good starting condition for such surgery. A body lift operation is also feasible in older age, but everything has its sensible limits. Clarification should always be made in advance from a medical and ethical point of view.

Procedure
The most common technique, "prone position-back position," is always performed when the outer sides of the thighs do not hang extremely. This technique gets its name because we operate on you first in the prone and then in the supine position. So you will be rotated on the operating table during surgery.

In the alternative technique, the "side-to-side supine position," you are first transferred to the left, then to the right, and in the last step to the back, in order to get good access to the outer sides of the thighs at all times. Whether we start on the left or right side is irrelevant.

Common to both techniques is a marking of the incisions before the operation on the ward. Different incision patterns are possible. Here, the steepness and positioning of the height of the scar resulting after the operation can vary depending on the body constitution. As with the abdominoplasty, the marking is done in the standing and lying positions.

We prefer incisions that are as deep as possible in order to be able to conceal the scars well. The deep horizontal incision, just above the mons pubis, runs to either side towards the anterior iliac spine (the upper, lateral pelvis) or slightly lower and then runs as an arc backwards to the upper buttock interfold area. This is where the two meet, creating a circular lift. As with other surgeries, up to a certain degree, we can agree on your personal wishes as to where the scar should be positioned.

After arriving in the operating room, the general anesthesia is induced as for body lift surgery partial anesthesia or local anesthesia is not an option. A bladder catheter is then placed, which, depending on the hospital, will remain in place for a few days postoperatively. Because of its disadvantages (increased risk of urinary infection), other centers do not use a bladder catheter. For your information, a urinary catheter should be placed whenever surgery lasts longer than 3–4 h so that the bladder does not overfill and is continuously emptied. Through the bladder catheter, the anesthesiologist can control and manage the fluid balance and thus the body's liquid inflow and outflow under anesthesia.

Now the positioning of your body for the operation takes place on the operating table. This is where the two techniques now differ. In the "prone position-back position" technique, you will be turned onto your stomach for the first step of the operation. The back, buttocks and the lateral flanks, and partially the outer thighs are tightened . In the "lateral side-back position" technique, you will first be positioned in a right or left side position and fixed in place with special supports. In this technique, the first step is to tighten the flanks, especially the outer sides of the thighs, and half of the back and buttocks.

With both techniques, only an upper buttock lift is performed. This means that there is no tightening in the area of the buttock folds. The soft tissues of the "upper buttock lift," that is, the skin-soft tissue excess that is normally discarded (resected), can be used for buttock augmentation. What this concerns, your plastic surgeon will explain the advantages, disadvantages, and options. The cost of buttock augmentation is your own responsibility.

A buttock lift in the area of the gluteal fold is to be distinguished from the upper buttock lift and would have to be applied for as such or taken over by a personal contribution. Information on the buttock lift can be found in Sect. 4.5.

After the skin incision, the excess skin soft tissues are detached and removed until sufficient tightening is achieved. As with the thigh lift, it is also important with the body lift that the detached soft tissues are firmly fixed to the body at so-called anchor points so that the wounds are not torn apart when you stand, the tightening effect is lasting and the scars do not widen.

In addition to the anchor sutures, we use also internal sutures to achieve long-term tightening. For this purpose, we use threads to tightly suture the fat fascia (connective tissue layer of firm tissue within the fat tissue) to create a stable situation and tightening. Only with a stable suture of the fat fascia, a body lift is possible at all. Otherwise, there is a risk that the tissue will tear apart when the patient stands up.

After suturing the fat fascia, the wound is closed with a deep and superficial skin suture using self-dissolving suture material. A temporary dressing is applied and you are repositioned. Two to four drains are inserted in the flank and back areas, and two drains are usually inserted in the abdomen. A total of four to six drains are thus placed.

In the "side lateral supine" technique, repositioning to the opposite side takes place and the same steps are performed as on the previously operated side. In the third step of this technique and in the second step of the "prone position-back position" technique, repositioning to the supine position takes place, and the body lift is completed on the anterior torso wall. Exactly the same steps are now performed as in an abdominoplasty, which, if you are interested, can be read about in the guide "Reconstructive surgery after massive weight loss." In principle, many different incision designs are possible for abdominoplasty. Therefore, the positioning of the incision and the resulting scar does not follow a fixed scheme but is individually adapted to the current conditions.

After repositioning on the back and redrafting the operative field, the skin incision is made in the area of the pubic hair, continuing towards the sides until the incision meets the scars from the back–buttock flank lift. The surrounding tissue is now separated from the abdominal muscles in a headward direction toward the belly button. Arriving at the belly button, it is incised with its skin portion and remains at its blood supply from the blood vessels from the abdominal cavity. The detachment of the skin and subcutaneous tissue continues headward toward the sternal notch.

Now it's time for the internal tightening: The straight abdominal muscles are paired and both run in a sheath ("rectus sheath"). The rectus sheath in turn connects the two straight muscles to each other via a layer of connective tissue. The muscles are usually widely separated, causing instability of the anterior trunk wall, and outward protrusion of the internal organs. This protrusion is brought together and sutured in the following step. This pushes the organs back into the abdominal cavity and results in internal shaping with a waistline. Local anesthetic is introduced into the suture area of the rectus sheath so that you feel as little pain as possible after the operation.

We then tighten the excess areas. For this purpose, the operating table is placed in a hip flexion position so that the upper and lower wound edges approach each other and we can remove as much tissue as possible and achieve a good tightening effect. The excess is removed and two drains are inserted. Don't be concerned: removing the drains can be a bit uncomfortable, but it is not painful. Wound closure begins with the so-called quilting sutures, where the detached abdominal wall is fixed to the abdominal wall from cranial to caudal closing the dead space created during initial skin detachment. In this way, we avoid one of the most common complications, seroma formation. In addition, the tension on the wound margin is reduced because the traction forces are distributed, which has a positive effect on wound healing and scarring. When the belly button is reached, its new position is decided upon. After incising the skin and subcutis, the belly button is delivered and sutured at this level with resorbable sutures.

The wound margin is closed over several layers. The fat fascia is again sutured under slight tension with resorbable sutures, thus achieving a stable situation on the one hand and an indirect tightening of the inner thighs on the other. This indirect thigh lift sounds better than it actually is. It results in a rather light tightening effect, which cannot be compared in any way with a direct tightening (with an incision directly above the thigh). Ask your attending physician specifically for examples using photos where indirect tightening of the inner thighs can be seen. This will give you a better idea of how much can be achieved with indirect thigh lift surgery.

Wound closure is now performed by deep and superficial skin suturing with self-dissolving sutures. The belly button is sutured with either self-dissolving or non-self-dissolving sutures, depending on the preference of the clinic where you are treated. We tend to use non-self-dissolving sutures in this area and remove the sutures after 12–14 days. We have had a very good experience with this. Afterward, staple plasters are applied to the wounds, undressed compresses are fixed over them and the compression suit is put on.

The operation time is between 2.5 and 5 h depending on the effort and planned additional operations.

The question always arises whether a T-cut (fleur-de-lis) in the area of the abdomen or back is possible during a body lift. It is possible, but not always necessary because through circular tightening the tissue excess can also be well redistributed. So it depends on what the initial conditions are and what is necessary.

After a body lift, a compression suit must be worn consistently day and night for at least 8 weeks. In Fig. 4.12a possible result of a body lift can be seen.

You will lie on your back in a bent position after the body lift surgery. We call this "stepped bed positioning ." This relieves the pressure on the suture. In principle, you may get up on the day of the operation, although only very few people do so. On the second day at the latest, you should mobilize yourself with help and, as soon as you are confident, on your own. The more successful this is, the faster the recovery process will be and many risks (such as the risk of thrombosis) will be significantly reduced.

When you initially stand up, you can only walk bent over because of the tension on your abdomen. Do not try to stand up against the pain, you might tear sutures and can cause the wound to open. You will notice on your own that, you will be able to progressively resume the upright position as each day passes. After the first to third week, you are expected to walk straight again. The inpatient hospital stay lasts between 3 and 7 days.

After the operation, you should try not to sneeze or push into the abdomen during solid bowel movements. If you still cannot avoid this, you should protect and counterpress the abdominal muscles with your two hands so that the inner suture on the straight abdominal muscles does not tear. The inserted drains are usually removed in the inpatient course if conveying not more than 25 ml/24 h.

In total, you should take it easy for 6–8 weeks. In our experience, you will be unable to work for at least 4 weeks, more likely 6 weeks. The incapacity to work can

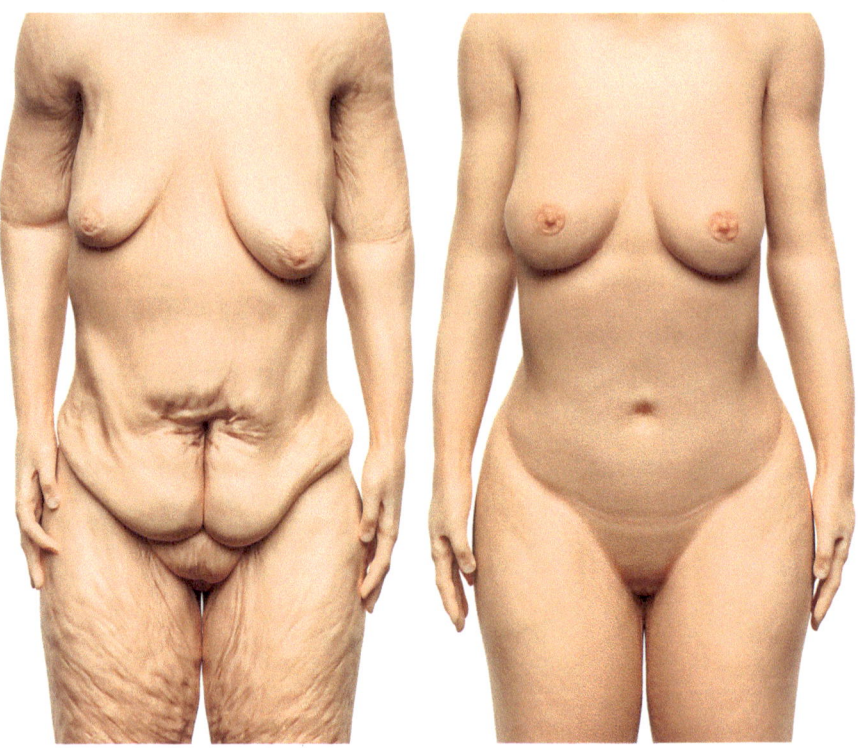

Fig. 4.12 Example of a result after circular body lift

be extended to 12 weeks in complicated cases, depending on the healing and recovery process. Likewise, you should not lift objects weighing more than 15 kg for 8–12 weeks so that the sutures of the internal tightening (rectus suture) do not tear. Light physical activities can be done from the second week, swimming—provided all wounds have healed—after 6–8 weeks. Jogging is allowed after 8 weeks at the earliest.

The scars should be blow-dried after showering or bathing. Once all wounds have healed, you can massage them with silicone gel one time a day for scar treatment.

Complications and Risks
With the body lift, as with all lifting operations, there are risks. Due to the prolonged operation time, the risks during the operation are higher than in other operations. These include blood loss (with the risk of administration of blood products), nerve or skin damage through positioning on the operating table, risk of venous thrombosis and hypothermia resulting in a prolonged recovery period after the operation. In addition, with a body lift you have a much larger wound area and also wound suture, so you also have a higher risk of wound healing problems in the suture area, accumulation of wound fluid, widened scars, and asymmetries.

Additional Information about Treatment

Zaher Jandali, Benedikt Merwart, and Lucian Jiga

5.1   Possibilities and Limits of Plastic Surgery

All planned surgeries will certainly be stressful and drain your strength, but in the end, it will be worth it. A new attitude towards life, with less or even no pain and a new self-awareness, awaits you.

> "I never thought I would be able to live such a life free of complaints."
> "All of a sudden, I can maintain my weight."
> "It's insane how my body shape has changed for the better."

These are all typical statements from patients who have already undergone treatment.

As different as your medical history and your own disease are, so are your expectations as patients seeking treatment. From our point of view, most patients have the realistic projection of the results to be expected (pain and aesthetics) after surgical treatment. However, a small percentage of patients have expectations that are too high and an even worse, a pathological perception of their own body image and what could be achieved through surgery. Like most others, you the reader, have realistic expectations on what can be achieved through surgery in terms of the goals can be reached. However, we can only determine these together with you during your consultation.

Z. Jandali (✉) · B. Merwart · L. Jiga
Department of Plastic, Aesthetic, Reconstructive and Hand Surgery, Evangelical Hospital Oldenburg, Oldenburg, Niedersachsen, Germany
e-mail: dr@jandali.de

5.2   How to Find the Right Doctor?

The question on how to find the right doctor seems anecdotal at first glance. However, it is a question not easy to answer. Liposuctions are performed by physicians with very different training backgrounds.

In Germany, medical studies last 6 years. After graduation, we receive a license to practice medicine. From this moment on, a german physician is basically allowed to do everything from heart surgery to cesarean sections up to aesthetic surgery. This means that the license to practice medicine alone qualifies him, at least on paper, to do anything he feels able to do without even considering a residency program in a certain field of interest. This until a complication arises, at which moment, his skills are measured directly against the standard of a consultant in that field.

As a consequence, many physicians from different specialties, including many without residency training, are involved in cosmetic surgery and liposuction. We have seen this procedure performed by internists, general surgeons, gynecologists, dermatologists, oral and maxillofacial surgeons, even orthopedics, and trauma surgeons . Among all these physicians, as in any medical field, there are doctors with very good skills but also ones with a lower amount of experience. But the question that arises is: Is there a specialty in which physicians are more likely than others to be confronted with these techniques during training and thus learn to deal with the entire ray of their possible complications on a frequent basis?

Yes, this specialty exists. With a very high degree of probability, plastic and aesthetic surgeons are the ones with arguably the highest experience in this field. In contrast, there are physicians who simply call themselves "cosmetic surgeons ." This is where the wheat is often separated from the chaff because the term "cosmetic surgeon" is a non-protected term that any doctor can adopt as a title—even if he or she has not completed any residency or ever held a scalpel in his or her hand. That's a bit of a problem in many health systems in Europe. Unfortunately, many patients, being blinded by the outstanding design of an office, the warm words and the nice manner can fall into a scenario possibly exposing them to serious complications. But honestly, what good is a nice doctor with a nice office, who will have serious decisional issues in handling a complication after one of his surgeries?

In Germany, the title "specialist in plastic and aesthetic surgery," can only be acquired by physicians who undergo training (residency), meet certain minimum requirements to register for an examination, and successfully pass this exam.

In plastic and aesthetic surgery, the residency takes 6 years of training. During this time, skills, including certain surgeries, must be learned and practiced. In this regard, the plastic and aesthetic surgery residency is the only residency in which liposuction is required in a high number. Otherwise, admission to the examination is not possible . In addition, the instructor must issue the trainee doctor with a so-called specialist certificate for the subject and thus also vouches with his name for competence that has been imparted.

▶   Look for the specialist designation "Plastic and Aesthetic Surgery."

In addition to performing liposuction, there is also training in the management of complications, such as corrective surgery. The treatment of complications is another key difference from other specialties and should be included in the decision-making process as well. Choosing an experienced plastic surgeon lays the foundation for a successful operation, but no doctor can guarantee freedom from complications. Complications can happen with any surgeon, even a plastic surgeon. We, too, have gone through many complications with our patients; yet, all have successfully accomplished the treatment, in the end,. As plastic surgeons dealing with complications and being able to correct them so as to provide an acceptable result for the patient in spite of "all odds" is our second nature. It is important to understand that complications do happen to all of us surgeons. Should you hear the statement that there are no complications for a certain surgical procedure, we strongly advise you to look for another doctor. While it is important to be open to your successes, admitting your complications and what you have learned from these, is the only way to warrant your progress as a doctor and offer rewarding therapy to your patient.

Are you currently on the lookout for a physician and an appointment? We recommend you to search for a colleague on the official website of society for plastic, reconstructive, and aesthtic surgery in your country (In Germany, this society is called "Deutsche Gesellschaft der Plastischen, Rekonstruktiven und Ästhetischen Chirurgen e.V."—DGPRÄC).

If you are in Germany, once you have found a suitable doctor when making the appointment ask whether he or she is also licensed by the health insurance. If your concern is a medically justified treatment (e.g., suffering from painful lipedema), you will only be able to get your treatment covered by your health insurance, if your physician has this special license. Otherwise, you would have to cover the costs of all appointments and treatment yourself.

It is important that you feel comfortable with the doctor treating you and that you trust the doctor. If this is not the case after the first appointment, a second opinion with a colleague is recommended. In any case, obtaining a timely opinion is a very sensible thing to do if there are still unanswered questions or uncertainties.

▶   All plastic surgeons who belong to the German Society of Plastic, Reconstructive, and Aesthetic Surgeons (DGPRÄC) can be found on the website www.dgpraec.de. Here you can conveniently obtain contact details of the nearest plastic surgeon via a search mask using your postal code.

▶   Personally, we can also strongly advise you to see experienced specialists in plastic and aesthetic surgery and not to turn to doctors practicing outside this field.

5.3   Presentation to the Plastic Surgeon

You are certainly eagerly awaiting the first appointment with the plastic surgeon and hope that the visit will initiate the process of lipedema treatment. Of course, seeing a plastic surgeon is a crucial step for many. This book was written to make your appointment informative and productive. If the answers have not been already clarified during the initial workup, we recommend asking the physician a clear set of questions from the checklist below (Table 5.1).

Although almost all plastic surgeons probably deal with liposuction and skin-tightening surgery for lipedema, as in any mixed group, there are specialists in one or the other. There are two to three easy ways to find out if a doctor is familiar with lipedema. The easiest way is to ask your support group or other patients, how many cases of lipedema are treated by a particular doctor. Further information on the doctor, the surgery, aftercare, and overall result are also important to make the right decision.

You can also clarify this point when making an appointment on the phone or over the Internet by simply asking, "Do you specialize in treating lipedema?" If so, you are correct, if not, you should contact another colleague.

Table 5.1 Checklist for the presentation to the plastic surgeon

Before the appointment	
Choosing the right doctor	Search the website at www.dgpraec.de
	Inquire in advance if the attending physician is a plastic surgeon
	Ask on the phone if the plastic surgeon also performs liposuction and tightening surgeries
	Ask if the doctor also performs liposuction at the expense of the health insurance (if your concern is to apply for the surgery to the health insurance)
	Sort through your medical records and the timeline of your medical history. Make notes
In the appointment	
Questions from the doctor to you	How long have you been suffering from lipedema?
	What was the course?
	In overweight patients: Failed diet attempts? Bariatric surgery? When, what, where?
	Weight reduction: If yes, how long has the current body weight been maintained? Preexisting conditions before and after weight reduction?
	Presentation to the vascular surgeon?
	Compression stockings?
	Lymphatic drainage?
	Family burden?
	Medication?
	Allergies?
	Do you do sports?
	Do you smoke?
	Family history (hereditary diseases, occupation, children)?
	What bothers you?
	Which body regions are affected?
	Are there medical reasons for the treatment or are only aesthetic (external) aspects in the foreground?
	What do you wish for?

Table 5.1 (continued)

Before the appointment	
Your questions to the doctor	Which operations are recommended in which technique?
	How do the operations proceed?
	How long is the expected hospital stay?
	How long will you be unable to pursue your work?
	How is it regulated with compression garments and how with secondary care?
	What complications can occur and how are they treated?
	Is there an intensive care unit in the hospital?
	Where and how is the aftercare of the operations?
	Will there be any costs for you?
	What costs will you incur if the procedure cannot be covered by health insurance? Is VAT included in the price?
	If the surgery is covered by health insurance, are there additional procedures that are not covered by health insurance but would significantly improve the final result, such as liposuction adjacent to the region?
After the appointment	
Administrative	Affirm the medical necessity of your tightening surgery by obtaining certificates from co-treating primary care physicians and vascular physicians
	Send the plastic surgeon's certificate together with your application and the certificate of the co-treating physicians to your responsible health insurance company

▷   Introduce yourself to a specialist.

A typical plastic surgeon interview starts with a friendly and open greeting. You don't need to be flustered; it will be a casual open conversation, and the doctor will take plenty of time with you. The doctor will briefly introduce himself and then ask why you are seeking his help.

The classic question would be, "What brings you to us?" or "What can I do for you?" You're already in the middle of the conversation. You should share a brief summary of your medical history. You may also have the information written down sorted on a small piece of paper. This should be followed by a discussion of preexisting conditions and current illnesses. What illnesses existed and what illnesses currently exist? Have there been any surgeries in your medical history? Finally, briefly discuss the medications you are currently taking and any allergies you may have.

Do you exercise regularly? Do you smoke, and if so, for how many years and how many cigarettes per day? Your family history also plays a role: Do you live alone? Do you have children? What is your profession? Are there any hereditary diseases in the family?

Now it is time to go into the actual reason for your appointment. You should go into detail about your complaints: on the one hand, what bothers you purely physically (physically) and, of course, what bothers you from your purely aesthetic point of view. It is important that at this moment you attach an honest and comprehensive description of your physical discomfort.

The interview is followed by an examination so that the doctor can obtain an actual picture. This is where your subjective perception comes together with our objective assessment. Often what is described by the patient matches what we see, but sometimes it does not. If a medical justification cannot be derived or attested, it is possible to apply to the health insurance company for reimbursement, but this is very rarely successful. In case of a refusal by the health insurance company, you have the option to bear the costs yourself. During the examination, we obtain an overall view and, of course, also examine the individual areas of the body.

After summarizing your medical history, the complaints, and the examination findings, an individual therapy plan is drawn up. Likewise, the operations that are being considered should be explained and further procedure clarified. Ask to be shown before-and-after pictures that resemble your body so that you can get a realistic idea of the possible results. Do not compare yourself to before-and-after pictures of sufferers who have a significantly different overall body shape than you.

Index

A
Abdominoplasty, 191
Adjustable gastric band, 102
Anaesthesia, 136
Apparatus intermittent compression
    (AIK), 109
Aspect dilution, 127
Aspect tumescent solution, 127

B
Body-contouring, 123
Body mass index, 64, 65
Body-sculpting, 123
Bottom-up, 161
Bruises, 142
Buttock lift, 181, 190

C
Calorie turnover, 38
Capillary permeability, 24
Circular lower body lift, 192
Circumference, 67, 68
Complex surgical treatment, 111–113
Compression garment, 142
Compression therapy, 79
Conservative measures, 98
Cosmetic surgeons, 200
Cost absorption, 167

D
Dry technique, 118
Duodenal switch, 105, 106

E
Energy transfer, 179
Estrogen, 12
Exercise therapy, 111

F
Fat apron removal, 191
Fat distribution, 36
Fatty acid synthesis, 8
Fibrose, 13
Fluid balance, 141

G
Gastric bypass, 103
Ghrelin, 16

H
Harris-Benedict formula, 39
Helium plasma beam, 180
Hemoglobin (Hb), 128
Hyperplasia, 9, 21
Hypertrophy, 9, 21

I
Insulin, 15

K
Kinderwunsch, 165

© Springer Nature Switzerland AG 2022
Z. Jandali et al. (eds.), *Lipedema*, https://doi.org/10.1007/978-3-030-86717-1

L
Leptin, 16
Lipedema, 1, 90, 95–97
    adipose tissue, 5, 6
    autologous fat grafting, 171, 172, 174–176
    capillary permeability, 24, 25
    causes, 4, 24
    chronic-progressive, 31, 32
    classification, 48–50, 52–56
    complaints, 44–48
    complex physical therapy, 107, 108,
        110, 114
    cost absorption, 167–170
    diagnosis, 56, 57, 59, 64
    edema, 23, 29
    energy consumption, 43
    energy intake, 40, 42, 43
    estrogen, 12, 13
    fat swelling, 2
    function, 7, 8
    ghrelin, 16
    history, 3
    imaging diagnostics, 63
    individual therapy plan, 114, 115
    inspection, 60
    insulin, 15
    leptin, 16
    lymphatic interaction, 21
    microvascular disruption, 21
    obesity, 32, 33, 35, 37
    obesity-associated lymphedema, 27
    orthostatic edema, 26
    pain, 30, 31
    palpation examination, 61
    progesterone, 14
    science, 9–11
    structure, 7, 8
    treatment, 166, 167
    uncontrolled fat tissue proliferation, 21
    waist-to-height ratio (WHtR), 67
    weight stabilization, 98–103, 105,
        108, 111
Lipoaspirat, 123
Lipohypertrophy, 17, 18, 20
Lipolymphedema, 91
Liposuction, 85, 86, 115, 116, 129
    aftercare, 140, 141, 143–145
    aspect bleeding, 128
    aspect dilution, 127
    classic liposuction, 120
    complex-operative therapy plan, 160
    consequences, 150–156, 158

laser-assisted liposuction, 123
    long-term prospects, 146, 147
    plans, 164–165
    power assisted liposuction, 122
    preparations, 130–134
    procedure, 137–139
    quantity specification, 125, 126
    safe suction volume, 126
    SRL, 161
    techniques, 117–119
    time expenditure, 129
    volume, 123
    water jet assisted liposuction, 121
Lymphatic capillaries, 70
Lymphatic drainage, 141
Lymphedema, 88–91, 93
    anatomy, 69, 70
    causes, 73, 74
    clinical appearance, 75, 76
    conservative therapy, 78, 81
    diagnosis, 76, 77
    primary lymphatic organs, 70
    secondary lymphoid organs, 70, 73
    surgical therapy, 81–85
Lymphocytes, 70
Lymphoid organs, 70

M
Macro fat, 172
Manual lymphatic drainage (MLD),
        78, 109
Medical indication, 177
Micro fat, 174
Microangiopathy, 26
Mini bypass, 105

N
Narrow tube, 103

O
Obesity, 32, 33

P
Painkiller, 140
Palpation, 89
Phlebo-lymphedema, 91
Plastic surgeon
    limits, 199

possibilities, 199
presentation, 202–204
right doctor, 200, 201
Plastic surgery, 199
Power assisted liposuction, 122
Power metabolism, 39, 40
Primary lymphatic organs, 70
Progesterone, 14
Psyche, 44

Q
Quantity specification, 125

R
Ralf way, 101, 102
Rehabilitation treatment, 111

S
SADI-S, 106
Scars, 144
Skin care, 81
Skin flaps, 177
Skin irritation, 177
Skin lesions, 89
Stemmer's sign, 61
Stepped bed positioning, 197
Systematic regional liposuction, 161

T
Thigh lift, 181
complications, 185
procedure, 181, 183, 184
risks, 185
Thrombosis, 155
Tightening methods, 179
Tissue removal/debridement, 86
Torso wall, 192–194
complications, 198
procedure, 194–197
risks, 198
Triflow, 159

U
Ultrasound-assisted liposuction (UAL), 122
Ultrasound examination, 63
Upper arm lift, 186, 187
complications, 189, 190
procedure, 188, 189
risks, 189

V
Visual analog scale, 59

W
Waist–hip ratio (WHR), 65